the ultimate baby
and toddler q&a

By Netmums and available from Headline

the ultimate baby and toddler q&a

Your 50 most common questions answered

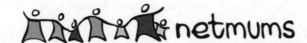 netmums

Parents and experts share advice and experience

with Hollie Smith

headline

First published in 2012
by HEADLINE PUBLISHING GROUP

1

To avoid the awkward use of 'he/she' or 'his/her' throughout the book, we have used
alternate male and female examples in each chapter.

The purpose of this book is to present solutions that have worked for other parents.
Readers will need to make their own choices, as they know their child and their
environment best, but must also bear in mind guidelines from the government
and other advisory organisations. The author and publisher cannot take
responsibility for any person acting as a result of the information
contained in this book.

Some of the Netmums contributors' names have been changed to protect their privacy.

Cataloguing in Publication Data is available from the British Library

ISBN 978 0 7553 6110 6

Typeset in 11/14.5pt Clearface by Palimpsest Book Production Limited,
Falkirk, Stirlingshire

Printed and bound in the UK by
Clays Ltd, St Ives plc

Headline's policy is to use papers that are natural, renewable and
recyclable products and made from wood grown in sustainable forests.
The logging and manufacturing processes are expected to conform
to the environmental regulations of the country of origin.

HEADLINE PUBLISHING GROUP
An Hachette UK Company
338 Euston Road
London NW1 3BH

www.headline.co.uk
www.hachette.co.uk

Contents

Introduction

Bringing up children is constantly challenging. But there'll never be as many questions in your mind as there are during the baby and toddler years. Feeding, teething, development, sleep (to name but a few): the list of issues thrown up in this first phase of parenthood seems endless.

Unfortunately, as the cliché goes, babies don't come with instructions. New parents have to seek out the answers to their questions as best they can. Which is where the *Ultimate Baby and Toddler Q&A* comes in. Having canvassed a group of Netmums to find out exactly what the most common quandaries are during this period, we came up with a comprehensive list of fifty. It includes all the old chestnuts ('When will he sleep through the night?' and 'When should I start weaning?' for example), but I'm proud to say it also tackles the thornier subjects, too. (For instance: 'Is breast-feeding supposed to be this difficult?' and 'Will our sex life ever be the same again?')

Of course, as the many and varied threads on the Netmums forums reveal, there's never one definitive answer to any question. Our books reflect that fact, which is why they include a mix of advice from a panel of down-to-earth experts (all of whom are also parents), and a wide range of opinions from the Netmums themselves. The result is a compendium of friendly, non-prescriptive guidance, which should help you through the tricky bits of the baby and toddler years, without laying down a whole load of 'rules' that on difficult days, you haven't a hope of sticking to.

The early years of parenthood can be wonderful. But they're even better with some help behind you.

Siobhan Freegard
Founder, Netmums

Meet the team

Hollie Smith is a freelance journalist and author of nine books about parenting, six of them written for Netmums. She's married and has two daughters, aged ten and seven. www.holliesmith.co.uk

Louise Cremonesini qualified as a nurse in 1993 and worked for five years in adult intensive care before training as a specialist children's nurse and spending ten years in paediatric intensive care at Great Ormond Street and the Royal Brompton hospitals. She has a BA (hons) degree in public health, and worked for five years as health visitor, first for Ealing Primary Care Trust and then Cambridgeshire Community Services. Now in her third year of an MSc programme in vulnerable children and families, she recently became a senior lecturer in children's nursing and health visiting at Northampton University. She is married to David and has a four-year-old daughter, Amelia.

Dr David Cremonesini studied medicine at Oxford University and St George's Hospital Medical School in London, and has been working in paediatrics since 1997. He spent two years at the John Radcliffe Hospital in Oxford where he developed an interest in respiratory paediatrics and allergy, and now works as a general paediatrician specialising in allergic and breathing problems in a hospital in Cambridgeshire.

Maggie Fisher qualified as a nurse in 1977 at The London Hospital, where she also completed a course on specialist and intensive care of the newborn, and worked in the neonatal intensive care unit. She has worked as a health visitor for 27 years in London and Hampshire, and ran a sleep support group for 15 years. She has a post graduate diploma in Promoting the Mental Health of Infants and Children and has contributed to a book about parenting in public health, as well as writing her own book about skill mix in health visiting and community nursing teams. Maggie is chair of Unite/ CPHVA (Community Practitioners' and Health Visitors' Association) Health Visitors' Forum and works for Netmums as a health visitor parent supporter. She lives in Hampshire and has three children, a 16-year-old daughter and sons aged 22 and 24.

Crissy Duff is a qualified Psychotherapeutic Counsellor and a member of the British Association for Counselling and Psychotherapy. She counsels both adults and children in her private practice as well as in schools, a local GP surgery and in the Occupational Health Department of her local borough council. Having been a popular member of the Netmums team since 2004, she now works as one of the site's parent supporters, counselling members with a wide range of problems. Crissy is married and has daughters aged thirteen and eleven and a son aged eight.

PART ONE: NEWBORN

1 How should I handle him?

Newborns can seem like the most vulnerable and fragile creatures on earth. It's not unusual to feel apprehensive about picking up, holding, cuddling, carrying, dressing and otherwise handling your little one at the start – especially if he's your first and you don't have much in the way of previous experience, or if he was born early and had a low birth weight. There are a few basic techniques to get to grips with and one or two rules to bear in mind when handling your baby. After that, it's just a matter of developing confidence. You'll soon get there, with a little practice.

Do be sure to pick up, hold and cuddle your newborn as much as he seems to need you to. It's the best way for you to get to know each other.

What the experts say

Louise says: What's important when picking up or holding your baby is keeping him close, so he can be reassured by the feel of your heartbeat and your warmth. Try to hold him confidently, firmly and securely, so he'll know he's in safe hands. Don't grip too tightly, though, as it could be uncomfortable for him.

When picking him up from a lying down position, slide one hand under his hand and neck, and the other underneath his bottom before scooping him up and bringing him quickly in close to you.

Good carrying or cuddling positions to try at first are the traditional cradle hold, where you support his head in the crook of your arm, and the shoulder hold, where you have him against your chest, his head nestling into your neck, with one hand supporting the back of his head and neck, and the other beneath his bottom or back. Another nice way to hold a newborn is facedown, along the length of your arm. This is particularly good for colicky babies because it puts a little pressure on their tummies and if you bob your arm gently up and down it can be soothing. (For more on colic see Question 15.) You need to be confident about this position, so perhaps it won't be the first thing you try, and it also helps to have a long, strong arm – so it's often popular with dads. Whatever hold you use, practise it sitting down first before trying to do it standing up or walking around, and most importantly of all, always make sure your baby's head is supported. It's unlikely to cause any serious damage if it lolls momentarily – and we've all been there – but it won't be comfortable for him. Likewise, if you carry your newborn round in a sling, which lots of parents find is a good way to offer an unsettled baby comfort in the early weeks, make sure it's suitable for his age, as they don't all have effective head support.

Do be careful when walking around with your baby, especially when you're still getting used to carrying him. It may sound like obvious advice, but sadly it's not uncommon for tired new parents to take a tumble when holding their child. So don't wear crazy shoes, make sure floors and stairs are always clear of clutter, and hold on tight to the bannister when you're negotiating stairs. Slippery babies are particularly hard to handle, so take extra care when wet! (For more on baths, see Question 12.) It goes without saying that your baby should never be jiggled, shaken or thrown around in play.

When it comes to dressing and undressing him, bear in mind that many babies dislike this process. Make sure clothes are the right fit, have everything you need to hand, and avoid complicated outfits while you're still getting your technique sussed – simple sleep suits are your best bet at the start. Widen neck, arm and leg holes with your fingers, and scrunch up fabric: aim to manipulate the garment on to your baby, rather than the other way round! Like every other aspect of caring for him, it will come with experience.

Dr David says: There are no hard and fast rules about how you should hold a baby, but what is important is to support a baby's head when you're holding him or picking him up. He'll gradually gain enough strength over the course of the first five or six months to support his own head but until then it will be very floppy and will always need a supporting hand from you.

One other thing I'd say is, do be wary if you're sitting on a sofa or chair cuddling your baby whilst tired, or after having a drink. You could fall asleep and then you run the risk of crushing or suffocating him, or of him rolling off and falling to the floor.

Crissy says: Getting to grips with handling your newborn can feel like a risky business at first, and for most of us it does take a while to really get the hang of holding our baby with any degree of confidence. Having looked forward to cradling your baby in your arms it can be a huge shock to find yourself fretting that you might accidentally hurt him. Most mums feel a bit wobbly in the early days, but it really is a case of practice makes perfect. The good news is that although your little one is tiny and you do need to take care, babies are actually much tougher than they look.

It's really important that you do pick up and cuddle your baby lots! It will help foster an emotional intimacy and allows both parties to get better acquainted. After the warmth and security of the womb the world can be a scary place, and touch is an essential ingredient for healthy infant development. It can also help mums come to terms with the end of their pregnancy – many women miss the wonderful sense of closeness that feeling their baby moving inside them can bring. This often quite profound sense of loss can be difficult to identify, let alone put into words, and mums may keep these difficult emotions bottled up for fear of being judged as foolish or even selfish. As a new mum, you may be warned against picking up your baby 'too much', the suggestion being that it could spoil him and make him needy and overly dependent. Well, to put it bluntly, you can't spoil a newborn! Of course he's dependent on you and he needs you to help him feel better. So don't feel guilty for sneaking that extra cuddle or soothing him in a baby sling. As he grows, having a strong and trusting attachment to his mum will give your baby the confidence and security he needs to go solo, knowing you're always on hand should he need you. So hold your baby while you still can, because before you know it he'll be crawling and you'll be struggling to keep up.

What the netmums say

Handling with care

For the first week or so, I was too nervous to even try picking my first baby up. She just seemed so fragile and I thought I might split her in two. My other half had to scoop her up and bring her to me for feeds and cuddles. Once she'd put on a few pounds – and I'd ceased to be such a nervous wreck – it was fine.
Lorna from Milton Keynes, mum to Sadie, fourteen months

When my son was born I was quite nervous of holding him because I hadn't really been around small babies very much before. I needn't have worried though; it felt quite instinctive the first time I picked him up, as if it was something I'd always been able to do but just never done. Babies are a lot more robust than we think.
Cathy from Reading, mum to Danny, two

I was fine holding my little girl, but terrified of dressing her! I kept thinking I would hurt her. I didn't though (I hope!). I remember being worried when I was pregnant that it wouldn't come as naturally as it did. Don't be afraid to ask for help if you need it.
Caroline from Alton, mum to Molly, eight months

It all came pretty naturally to me, to be honest. I wasn't at all worried about picking her up, but then I had had experience of babies previously, as I had a nephew and nieces. My husband was more nervous, and looked a bit cack-handed at first, but it didn't take him long to get the hang of it. I think it was just a confidence thing with him.
Esther from Hockley, mum to Charlotte, eleven, and Lauren, nine

I wasn't really worried about picking my son up, but undressing and dressing him worried both me and my other half, in case we hurt his neck or head.
Clare from Doncaster, mum to Connor, eighteen months

For the first twelve hours of his life, I was too scared to even touch my little man. He was born at thirty-one weeks and weighed 3.5 lbs – even compared to the other babies in the NICU at the time, he was tiny. My boyfriend felt the same. We just had to put aside our worries and, thankfully, staff were on hand to help. I felt like I should just 'know' how to hold him, feed him and dress him, but now I've made peace with the fact that my fears were all natural given our circumstances and we were simply coping with things as best we could.
Pam from Arklow, mum to Ruairí, seven months

I've had five babies (the smallest being 6 lb 6.5 oz, and the biggest 7 lb 13 oz), and everytime, I've worried that I'm going to hurt them when I get them dressed. But I never have.
Gemma from Poole, mum to Johnathan, nine, Keith, seven, Xander, three, Corbin, two, and Logan, five months

I wasn't nervous about holding my little one while I was at the birth centre, even though he was only 5 lb 12 oz at birth. But I was nervous about it when I got home, when the three of us were completely alone. I think I rang my mum every hour asking questions about what I should do next! For me, holding him and caring for him didn't come naturally. It took a couple of weeks for me to recover enough so I was confident to look after him, then it became easier. Now everything is second nature.
Clare from London, mum to Josh, six months

To be honest, it all came naturally with my firstborn and worry never really crossed my mind. I wasn't completely sure how to pick her up, hold her or dress her. But I just improvised!
Ellie from Poole, mum to Gina, twelve, Stewart, eight, and Julie, two

Oddly, I wasn't scared of picking up my first daughter, but with my second I was terrified! Perhaps it was because Megan was smaller and seemed more fragile than Chloe ever did.
Clair from Portsmouth, mum to Chloe, two, and Megan, four months

2 Is she supposed to sleep this much?

Lots of parents are surprised by how much their baby sleeps in the first couple of weeks after birth, but it's very normal – the average newborn spends between sixteen and twenty hours out of every twenty-four asleep. Because their tiny tummies need regular refuelling, they should in theory wake regularly for a feed, but sometimes they'll snooze for very long stretches which, in the daytime, can seem a little concerning. There's no need to fret, though. Newborns have yet to develop a functioning 'body clock', which means they can't tell the difference between day and night. For that reason, there probably won't be any clear pattern to her sleeping and waking for a while.

Unless you've been specifically advised by a health professional to wake her for feeds, there's no reason why you can't let her sleep as much as she seems to want to in the day. As for those frequent night-time wakings, there's little you can do about it in this early stage, apart from giving her whatever she needs in the way of feeding or comfort to drop off again. Do, however, make the most of your newborn's long daytime naps – and preferably not for catching up on housework or entertaining visitors, but to get some rest yourself.

What the experts say

Maggie says: It's absolutely normal for newborn babies to sleep loads in the first few weeks of life. It's because their 'circadian rhythms' have yet to settle – in other words, they don't have a developed body clock yet and so have no sense of what's day and what's night. Babies who've had difficult births can also spend a large part of their early days 'sleeping it off' and premmies tend to nap even more than is typical, probably because they have even more growing to do than those born full-term, and sleep is necessary for that.

Newborns will usually wake up at least every two to four hours for a feed, but sometimes they do sleep on even longer than that. Lots of parents wonder if they should wake their baby for food. It's best as a general rule *not* to wake her, otherwise you'll interfere with her natural sleep/wake rhythm – unless you've been advised otherwise by a health professional. She'll probably make up for any long stretches without milk by filling up when she does wake.

By around six to eight weeks your baby should start to take longer sleeps at night and smaller ones in the day, so it does settle into a more predictable and less anti-social pattern after a short time. You can help encourage this process right from the start by trying to differentiate between night and day: when you feed or change her at night, keep the lights low and keep things quiet and boring, and in the daytime, open the curtains, take her down-stairs, and spend lots of time talking and playing with her.

It's worth being aware of growth spurts, which can occur any time in the first few months, because during these periods, your baby's sleep requirements change and she may be snoozing even more than usual.

Other than that, all you can really do at this early stage is to go with the flow, and let her feed and sleep whenever she seems to need it. The truth is she's very likely to be all over the place in the first few weeks.

Dr David says: The amount of sleep that new babies need can sometimes be a bit worrying for new parents, but it's perfectly normal. It shouldn't normally be necessary to wake your baby up for a feed – unless you've been advised to for a specific reason, perhaps because your baby is a premmie, was small at birth, or is suffering from high levels of jaundice, which can make babies extra sleepy. As long as she's getting a good amount of milk in whilst she *is* awake, and there are no concerns over her size or growth, it should be fine to let her sleep as long as she wants. Unfortunately for tired new parents, lots of babies at this stage make up for any lack of feeding in the day by taking more at night instead. It's just the way it goes, I'm afraid – things will usually settle into a more civilised routine after the first few months!

Sleepiness *can* be an indication that a baby is poorly, but it's probably only a worrying sign if your baby suddenly becomes *more* sleepy than she's previously been and/or there are also other symptoms such as a high temperature present (see Question 26). If in any doubt at all, check with your midwife, health visitor or GP.

What the netmums say

Forty winks and more

My first was asleep all day and awake most of the night! I thought it wasn't natural but also assumed I should not wake a sleeping baby. By four months, though, things had balanced out and she was sleeping more at night, and for only a couple of hours during the day. My second also slept constantly at first, during the day. However, my third hardly slept at all, probably because there was so much going on around her, and was wide awake most of the time.
Ellie from Poole, mum to Gina, twelve, Stewart, eight, and Julie, two

For the first few weeks my son slept *all* the time and I was really worried about it. Then suddenly he woke up and stayed awake for about three bloody years! My advice would be to enjoy the peace and sleep while it lasts.
Jill from Berkhamsted, mum to Jay, seven

Chloe slept all the time as a newborn. I ended up waking her for feeds during the daytime, as she slept for hours on end, and I was worried she was missing out on milk. Megan is the same. Maybe I just have lazy babies?
Clair from Portsmouth, mum to Chloe, two, and Megan, four months

Even at the very start, my first daughter went to sleep at 6 p.m., woke at 9 a.m., and had two two-hour sleeps in the day. My second never slept – day or night – apart from an hour or so, here and there, until he was three. My third got day and night completely the wrong way round until he was about ten weeks old – then he slept from 8 p.m to 4.30 a.m., with just one sleep in the day for an hour. I guess all babies are different.
Claire from Reading, mum to Charlotte, twelve, Patrick, eleven, and Louie, six

When my eldest son was a newborn, he would only sleep when he was being held. I used to make myself a coffee, put on a good movie and let him sleep on my lap. Without sleep he became very grumpy, but he just wouldn't sleep on his own. My youngest was the opposite: he slept and slept. I remember being worried because he was hardly ever awake!
Irma from Oldham, mum to Damir, four, and Aydin, two

I was amazed at how much my first daughter slept in the early weeks. I was a bit neurotic then and would often go up to her crib and put my face close to hers just to make sure she was still alive! I know you're supposed to use the time to catch up on some sleep yourself, but I spent quite a bit of time just staring at her. With my second daughter I was more relaxed and could probably have used the time for some extra kip – if I didn't have an older child who was badly in need of a bit of attention!
Sharon from Stoke, mum to Mia, four, and Lily, two

Everyone says they tend to sleep lots at first, but even as a newborn my son never slept for long during the day. He'd only doze for an hour or two maximum in the first couple of weeks and even now, his naps are never more than an hour long. It would be nice if they were longer – I might get more done!
Helen from Sheffield, mum to Ryan, fifteen months

My son Kieran only ever used to sleep for half an hour at a time in the day, although he slept through the night from eight weeks. My daughter Livvy, on the other hand, was asleep for most of the

day, just waking for feeds and nappy changes. Her 'awake' time until she was three months old was between 8–11 p.m., when I really wanted her to be asleep! I didn't get a photo of her with her eyes open until she was three days old, and people always used to comment about how she was always asleep. I took her to the doctor in the end, who told me to make the most of it!
Natasha from Plymouth, mum to Kieran, four, and Livvy, two

3 How do I get started with breastfeeding?

If you plan to breastfeed your baby, your midwife should show you how – in fact, she'll want to make sure you both have the hang of it before you leave the hospital or birth centre. Getting into the most comfortable position possible and getting the 'latch-on' right are vital to getting started, and you'll almost certainly need a sympathetic professional to guide you as you find your way to the right technique.

Don't be afraid to ask for help if you're in any doubt about breastfeeding or how to do it. Your midwife or health visitor should be willing and able to give you support, but there should also be other sources of help via local breastfeeding counsellors, clinics, or relevant organisations such as the National Childbirth Trust (NCT) or La Leche League. There are also some good 'how-to' videos online. You'll need plenty of moral and practical support from your partner, too, and from at least one other reliable friend or relative when he returns to work – or if you are a lone parent. Breastfeeding can be hard work and time-consuming in the early weeks, so you need someone around to provide sustenance and encouragement.

However keen you are to feed your baby yourself, though, it's a good idea to remain realistic. Lots of mums find breastfeeding unexpectedly painful or tiring at first, and many give up before they'd planned. Taking things one day at a time is probably a good policy. (For more information about breastfeeding, see Question 11.)

What the experts say

Louise says: Getting your baby latched on right is key to happy breastfeeding. It can be tricky getting the perfect latch, but if you don't, you run the risk of getting seriously sore or cracked nipples. You want to get as much of the boob in his mouth as possible – if he's only just got the nipple in, that won't be right – with a minimum amount of areola (the darker skin around the nipple) visible below his bottom lip. His nose should be touching or close to the breast, but not squashed; his cheeks should be rounded, not sucked in; his chin should indent the breast; and his lower lip should be rolled outwards. Stop if it feels wrong, but don't just pull him off – insert your little finger into the corner of his mouth first, to break the suction. If your baby's sucking rhythmically and his ears are wiggling slightly, that's a sign you've got a good latch-on. You can also look at your nipple post-feed – if it seems misshapen that's an indication that you haven't. Do, however, be prepared for *some* pain while you're getting to grips with breastfeeding. Even if you *have* got the latch-on right, it may still hurt at the start of each feed.

Positioning is important, too. It should feel comfortable for you both. Always hold your baby close to you, with his head and body in a straight line, facing you, and make sure he's high enough that he doesn't have to strain upwards to get a good mouthful – his nose should be in line with your nipple. If the classic breastfeeding position isn't working for you at the start, try something different. The 'rugby ball' hold, when you tuck baby under your arm, is a good alternative, particularly if you've got large breasts. And if you're unwell or sore after a difficult birth, or just very tired, you may prefer to feed him whilst lying down. Using pillows for support can really help, whichever position you're in. And be careful not to push your baby's head when you're guiding him to your breast. It may feel to him as though he's being force-fed and that could really put him off.

There are great benefits for both mum and baby in breast-feeding, but it's not always plain sailing getting started. If you want to make a success of it, it's probably best not to have grand expectations. And don't hesitate to seek out help if you're struggling.

Maggie says: Getting your baby to the breast immediately after birth is the best possible way to establish breastfeeding. He'll often be in a quiet but alert state, which is ideal for feeding, and this really helps to get the colostrum (the nutrient-rich, creamy, first-stage breast milk) flowing. Skin-to-skin contact is also the nicest possible way for the two of you to get acquainted. Mums of SCBU babies (in special care units) may not have the same advantage, but having a picture of your baby in front of you and an electric pump should help to get the milk flowing.

Take it gently when offering your baby his first feeds. You sometimes see health professionals rather forcefully guiding a child into the breast, but it's better to help him use his instincts, by tickling the cheek nearest the breast. Babies have a 'rooting reflex' which means they will naturally seek out a breast and start suckling on their own.

It can take a while to get the latch-on right, which is why for so many mums it's painful at first, and you may need to practise. You might also have to try out different positions. But if you get these things right and you can get through the first few weeks the rest should be OK. It *will* come with time.

Breast milk is produced on a supply and demand basis, so it's really important from the start to put your baby to the breast whenever he seems hungry: it's the best way to keep on producing enough milk to keep feeding successfully. During growth spurts, which can crop up at any time, you'll probably find he wants to feed even more for forty-eight hours or so and if you're keen to keep going, you'll need to go with his demands.

Lots of people don't realise that a good calorie intake can help you to produce good-quality milk. Ideally, breastfeeding mums should eat three healthy meals a day, as well as several snacks, and make sure they get sufficient quantities of calcium, iron and vitamin C. You should be getting all that if you're eating a well-balanced diet with three meals a day and several healthy snacks in between. You may not have the time or energy to cook, so make sure someone else does so for you – or failing that, have plenty of ready-prepared, nutritious food ready to grab from the fridge. Get your partner to make you sandwiches before leaving for work, and if your mum or mum-in-law offers help, ask her to bring you hot food! Keeping well hydrated is important too, so drink plenty, particularly during feeds. An appropriate multivitamin supplement might be a good idea if your diet's falling short. In fact, it's recommended now that all breastfeeding mums aim to take 10 mcg of vitamin D daily, so you could look for a supplement that includes this. If you're on benefits, ask your HV (health visitor) about the Healthy Start scheme, as you may be entitled to free supplements.

Specialist help is all-important in getting breastfeeding started, and what's needed is someone who can sit with you and guide you in a relaxed environment. Your midwife or health visitor should be able to give you the support you need but, if not, trained breastfeeding counsellors can step in. The National Childbirth Trust is always a good starting point if you want to find one. There may also be help available at your nearest clinic, health centre or children's centre.

What the netmums say

Getting started with breastfeeding

My daughter was put on the breast as soon as I gave birth to her, which I feel helped a lot in establishing breastfeeding. I used Mothercare's own-brand nipple balm from the start, and never had any problems with cracked or sore nipples. If you want to breastfeed, do try – it's worth it. And never feel disheartened if you have to ask for help.
Claire from Portstewart, mum to Éabha, twenty months

On the first night at home with my tiny little daughter I was in a panic as I couldn't get her to latch on. After an upsetting night of trying, I rang a midwife at the hospital and she advised me to take all my clothes off from the waist up and lay her on my chest. I did this, and within seconds my baby daughter had latched straight on to my breast. She carried on feeding without problems until she was sixteen months old.
Lorraine from London, mum to Molly, five, and Evie, two

I had problems latching on and getting breastfeeding started with both of my babies. The main advice I would give is, get help. Find your nearest breastfeeding clinic, call a helpline, or, if you can afford it, pay for a visit from a lactation consultant. They're worth their weight in gold. Breastfeeding takes time and patience to get established.
Charlotte from Norwich, mum to Beatrice, three, and George, three months

Be prepared for your milk 'coming in' on the third or fourth day. It came as something of a shock when I work up with huge, hard, incredibly tender boobs that were spurting milk everywhere! It was harder than it had been to get him latched on – he really struggled to get his mouth round them.
Gemma from Watford, mum to Casey, ten months

I always knew I'd be a breastfeeding mum – after all, it's the most natural thing in the world, isn't it? But when my son was born, he just couldn't latch on properly. The birth centre midwives urged me to keep trying but by the following morning he still hadn't managed to feed. A breastfeeding support worker helped me get him latched on, and she then had to come in another three times as I just couldn't get it. In the end we tried feeding lying down, which seemed to work. Another support worker came to visit me at home twice and she helped me work out another position, which wasn't so antisocial. I kept going through those first difficult few days and I'm glad I did.
Clare from London, mum to Josh, six months

As a qualified breastfeeding peer supporter, I know that other mums who've successfully breastfed are the best resource for support when you're trying to get started. Look for help locally, at classes, clinics, or breastfeeding cafes, which provide a relaxed and friendly environment where you can get information and advice. The key is getting support early (ideally, before you've even given birth!).
Sam from Leicester, mum to Liam, two, and Lennon, fifteen months

I don't think all mums realise how much breastfed babies need feeding at first. With my first daughter, I didn't realise it was normal for a baby to have days when she fed all the time, and assumed I wasn't producing enough for her – so I ended up giving up after six weeks. Second time round I was determined to succeed for longer and I was better prepared. I also think a supportive partner who understands if breastfeeding is important to you, and does everything he can to help, is essential.

Angie from Arlesey, mum to Freya, six, and Tabitha, six months

First time, I was surprised how painful it was to start with. I did the National Childbirth Trust (NCT) breastfeeding course while pregnant, but there was no mention of pain! Maybe they think it'll put people off but personally I think I'd rather know that breastfeeding can be painful and difficult to start with *but* quickly gets a lot easier and – at least in my experience – enjoyable. After we got the hang of it, it was great. I felt really close to her. I'd recommend Lansinoh cream for sore nipples, and a breastfeeding cushion. I couldn't have done it without these, and the support of my partner. My NCT group was a great help, too.

Helen from Brockworth, mum to Rachel, two, and Charlotte, twenty-one months

4 Is it OK to bring her into bed with me?

Getting up in the dead of night to feed your baby can be an exhausting, cold and lonely experience. Who wouldn't be tempted to bring a little one into the warmth and comfort of the parental bed – particularly if you're breastfeeding and it makes perfect sense to do so lying down and half asleep? Yet most experts warn *against* bringing your baby into bed with you, because research suggests it's a risk to her safety. Government and NHS guidelines back the resounding message of the Foundation for Study of Infant Deaths (FSID), which is that the safest place you can put your baby to bed is in her own crib or cot, and, for the first six months of her life, to keep that cot in your room.

The fact is, though, that lots of parents *do* sleep with their baby. A few make a conscious decision to bedshare from the start, whilst for most it's just the way things work out – because it makes life easier or because it feels right at the time. So there's no definitive answer to this question. What's certain is that you should think carefully before bringing your baby into bed with you on a regular basis, and if you do, make sure you follow all the relevant guidelines so you're doing it as safely as possible. Safety issues apart, do also consider the possibility that later – when you're ready for your bed to be a child-free zone – your baby won't want to budge! And do make sure that bedsharing is a habit that your partner is happy to indulge. For some couples, it does not make for a harmonious set-up.

What the experts say

Maggie says: As a health visitor, I always advise parents against sleeping with their baby. Although the evidence is complex and ever-changing, it suggests that if you bedshare, your baby has a higher risk of cot death than if you put her to sleep in her own cot or crib in your bedroom. And bedsharing in conjunction with certain other factors is *definitely* a bad idea – you shouldn't bedshare, for example, if either you or your partner smokes, takes drugs or medication that could cause drowsiness, or has been drinking, or if your baby was premature or a low birth weight. Mums or dads who are very overweight are also warned against it, as are those who are 'excessively tired'. You shouldn't bedshare if you or your baby is poorly, or has a high temperature.

However, as a mum, I also know that it can feel very natural to have your baby in bed with you, particularly if you're breastfeeding. And research suggests that mums who bedshare tend to breastfeed for longer – so not all experts believe it's a bad idea. If you want to sleep with your baby, do your research and take all the safety recommendations to heart. So make sure you have a big enough bed, with a good, firm, snugly fitting mattress. Be certain your baby is not at risk of overheating – check your room temperature, don't overdress her and avoid heavy coverings. Also make sure her face isn't covered by your pillows or bedding, and that there's no chance of her falling out, or being trapped between mattress and wall. If you can, aim to sleep in a protective 'c-shape' round your baby, which will help to prevent her moving up and down the bed. Make sure she sleeps on her back, moving her gently back into position if she's been feeding on her side.

There is one other disadvantage to bedsharing, of course: your baby will probably come to rely on your proximity to settle. Teaching her the art of self-settling is the best thing you can do if you want her to eventually sleep through the night without any help from you. (For more on self-settling, see Question 21.)

One other thing I would stress is that whilst her own cot or crib is the safest place to settle your baby, that cot or crib should be kept close to your own bedside – at least, for the first six months, while the risk of cot death is at its highest. Lots of parents are keen to move their little one into a nursery, perhaps because they can be such noisy sleepers, but safe sleep research has concluded that – although it's not clear why – keeping your baby in your room with you is a crucial factor. Be very careful too, of falling asleep whilst feeding your baby in a chair or sofa. This is very risky, in case you drop her or crush her.

Dr David says: Sadly, about 300 babies still die suddenly and unexpectedly each year. Experts can't pinpoint a specific cause for cot death, but they do know that there are a number of factors that push the risk up. Bedsharing is one of them, and that's why medical professionals tend to advise parents against this practice. Certainly, it's a bad idea to bedshare when there are other risk factors at play, so if you do want to have your baby in bed with you, make sure you know what these are, and follow all the guidelines, as outlined by Maggie above. The risk for cot death is highest when a baby is two to three months old, with premature or low-birthweight babies especially vulnerable, and it falls sharply after six months, when it becomes very low. It's a fact that the safest place for your baby to sleep during her first six months is in her own cot or crib, in the same bedroom as you. Whatever you do, don't smoke, drink, or take drugs, and then share a bed with your baby. It's not worth the risk.

Crissy says: Whether it's a positive parenting choice or the last desperate resort of sleep-deprived mums and dads, there are plenty of convincing arguments in favour of bedsharing with your baby. Fans of co-sleeping feel that mum and baby sleep longer and more deeply and reckon that simply rolling over to breastfeed or comfort a newborn, rather than having to decamp to the next room, is less disruptive for all concerned. There's wisdom too in the suggestion that bedsharing offers busy working mums and dads a chance to make up for lost time with their baby. But these tempting advantages must be tempered by an awareness of the potential risks of co-sleeping. Parents should therefore take all necessary precautions and always aim to co-sleep as safely as possible. It's also worth bearing in mind the lifestyle concessions that having your baby in bed with you on a regular basis is likely to require. If you already share a bed with your partner, co-sleeping can make emotional and sexual intimacy difficult – which is why it's important that both mum *and* dad are happy with any such arrangement. Siblings, too, who are already struggling to adjust to sharing their parents with a new arrival, may feel jealous and excluded. So if it's not your first baby, the decision to bedshare requires careful consideration of what's best for the whole family.

What the netmums say

To bedshare, or not?

My daughter is a noisy feeder and to reduce my hubby's lack of sleep (he looked after her during the day while I slept, at first), I started off getting up at night and feeding her while sitting on the sofa. One night I realised, much to my alarm, that I'd dozed off and the next day decided to feed her sitting up in bed instead. Gradually I ended up lying on my side to feed her, and I still do this for night feeds. It means you get as much sleep as possible. Sometimes my daughter feeds while we are both asleep!
Amanda from Fleet, mum to Tabitha, nine months

I was adamant that I would not have our daughter in bed with us. I find the whole idea scary, the same as lying down on the sofa with her. I was so paranoid about it I wouldn't even breastfeed in the bed. My daughter has always been a fantastic sleeper. She's happy in her own space, and doesn't need her mummy or daddy to settle her.
Claire from Portstewart, mum to Éabha, twenty months

When I was pregnant I always said my baby would never sleep in bed with me. Alas, after three nights of her screaming in her Moses basket I gave in and took her in with me and she settled straight away. She's still in my bed now, at seven months. In a way I love it because of the closeness and the ease for breastfeeding, plus I'm a single mum, so it's nice for the cuddles. On the other hand, I regret it, as now she will not settle in her cot.
Sarah from Leicester, mum to Caitlyn, seven months

I didn't bedshare with my first. I think I was more patient and less tired. When my next one came along, he would go down in his own bed, but when he woke I would breastfeed him in bed and I couldn't get him out after that. My youngest would also usually spend the night in with us, but stopped at eight months. I used to think it was dangerous to co-sleep, but after reading up on it, I was convinced otherwise. I'm a deep sleeper but was always aware of my baby being next to me. My other half always had to sleep on the sofa if he'd been drinking.

Helen from Bude, mum to Amy, nine, Thomas, three, and Finlay, thirteen months

I always wanted to share our bed but my husband was worried about safety. So for the first few weeks I'd get up and down, and he'd be in and out of the cot (very difficult with infected stitches!). Then we realised we would all be happier sleeping together. So we bought a bed guard and we rolled up blankets to stuff in the gap between it and the bed. He slept in pyjamas and a Woombie [a snugly fitting sleeping bag] so he only needed a light blanket, whilst I always slept coverless to make sure he never got too warm. We still sleep together now and I intend to continue until he's ready to sleep alone.

Marianne from Uddingston, mum to William, twenty-two months

This is a no-no for me. We did with my first because I couldn't resist but once she was in, she had real trouble sleeping or getting to sleep without being in my room. So we agreed we were never going to do it again, for sanity's sake!

Ellie from Poole, mum to Gina, twelve, Stewart, eight, and Julie, two

I never did this with my son. He was in our room for a while, but never in our bed. I won't be co-sleeping with my next, either – as much as I love the idea – as I'm too scared that something will happen. It just unnerves me really, and I don't want to take the risk.

Isla from Beaconsfield, mum to Jordan, two

Like many others, I was adamant that I would not be bedsharing. My first was premature and I was so scared of losing her. However, she would not settle in the Moses basket, and I would fall asleep feeding her in bed. She would end up under the duvet some nights, which was worrying, so we moved her out and into a cot at three months where she's (mainly) been ever since. Our second daughter would sometimes come into bed with us but seemed happier to settle in her crib. She's now in a cot, sharing a room with her big sister, but sometimes comes into bed with us for a night feed. I'm a believer in doing what's best for you and I think anything that gives me more sleep to be able to function in the day is the best for me. I loved sharing a bed – but I love that my other half and I have now got it to ourselves again.

Louise from Sheffield, mum to Ella, two, and Grace, six months

Before my son was born I hadn't even heard of sharing the bed with a baby. We had the Moses basket all ready and set up next to the bed. However, the only way I could breastfeed my son was lying down. So from the first day he was home, we began sharing the bed, and we still do so now. I followed all the guidelines on safe co-sleeping, and haven't thought about it since.

Clare from London, mum to Josh, six months

For the first couple of weeks Joseph would only sleep on me or my other half, which was fine as we took it in turns to stay up while the other slept. However, when my other half went back to work I found I could get another few hours' sleep in the mornings by taking him out of his Moses basket and laying him on top of the covers next to me. He still likes this now but I don't let him do it too often as I don't want him to get used to it!

Laura from Aldershot, mum to Joseph, four months

I never planned on having babies in bed with me, but my eldest was so cuddly and would cry as soon as he was put down. Taking him into bed with us seemed the most natural thing to do and it allowed us all a chance for some decent sleep. He's four now and sleeps in his own bed most of the time, but does sneak in every now and again. My youngest, in contrast, has always liked his own space for sleeping and just wants to be left alone.

Irma from Oldham, mum to Damir, four, and Aydin, two

With our first two, I was always wary about co-sleeping and put them down in their Moses baskets, beside our bed. They were also both bottle-fed. Abigail, however, was breastfed and would not settle in her basket, so we decided to co-sleep. I follow the guidelines and make sure that she's not too hot and that she does not have any of our cover on her. I'm more relaxed third time round, and as she's breastfed it makes night feeds a whole lot easier. She's five months old now, and we still co-sleep – although I think my husband wishes we didn't!

Rachel from Staines, mum to Jake, five, Kyla, four, and Abigail, five months

5 Should his poo look like this?

You might be amazed, and perhaps concerned, about the appearance of your baby's poo – especially as it can so frequently change in colour, texture and quantity in the early weeks and months. From the sticky black stools at the start, to the lurid yellow hues that follow, not to mention the sometimes explosive nature of the stuff, it's not always obvious what a healthy baby's poo should actually look like. And on days when you find yourself wiping it off the back of his neck, or changing his sleep suit for the third time running, you might well wonder if it's normal!

Mostly there'll be no need for worrying, but all the same, it's worth keeping an eye on what you find in your baby's nappy, because it can be a useful indication that all's well – or not, as the case may be.

What the experts say

Louise says: Usually a baby's first poo will consist of, or contain, meconium – a black, tar-like mix of intestinal secretions, bile and swallowed amniotic fluid. Your midwife or doctor will want to make sure your baby's passed a poo of some sort within forty-eight hours of birth to be sure that his bottom and bowels are in working order. It's very sticky, but should come off fine with a little warm water and cotton wool, and perhaps a bit of plain soap if it's really caked on.

After that, you can expect a typical breastfed babe's poo to be very soft, with a seedy texture. Usually it's a mustardy colour

– I always describe it as a bit like chicken korma – but it can also be all sorts of shades either side of that, and it may well change from one day to the next for no obvious reason. Bottle-fed babies' poo, meanwhile, is more likely to be consistent in its colour and texture, fairly firm, and paler.

A change in the appearance of poo doesn't necessarily mean a problem – it could just be a minor reaction to something you've eaten, for example. Some parents baulk at poo that's very green, but even that's likely to be quite normal, in itself. As his mum, you'll get to know your baby's poo pretty well and you're very likely to notice if something's untoward.

Usually, breastfed babies will poo for Britain at first – typically after every feed, but after a while, it's not unusual for them to not have a poo for several days at a time. As they rarely become constipated, this shouldn't be a cause for worry. Bottle-fed babies are more likely to suffer from constipation and will generally poo every day or every other day, so if yours hasn't had a poo for three days or more, get it checked out with your health visitor or GP. (For more on constipation, see Question 24.)

As a general rule, seek medical advice if his poo looks unusual to you and it's accompanied with one or more other symptoms such as a temperature, fretfulness, vomiting or a rash. Some sorts of poo should be mentioned immediately to a health professional: if it has any red, black, or bloody bits in it, or if it's very pale or whitish in colour.

When your baby's poo is copious and runny, you might wonder if he's suffering from diarrhoea. In the case of a breastfed baby, it's almost certainly normal (and it would be pretty unusual as breastfed babies have lots of natural protection against gastrointestinal problems). If your baby is formula fed, diarrhoea is likely to be very different from the usual stuff, which will typically be quite firm. It will be distinctly watery and may contain mucus – and also, there's very likely to be other symptoms such as vomiting or weight loss.

The good news is that your baby's poo will usually settle down after a couple of months and become more regular. And there won't be nearly so much of it! ·

What the netmums say

Nappy talk

I remember being fascinated and a bit mystified by my newborn's poo, and how it changed colour each day! My brother has just had a new baby and there's actually a poo chart to colour in each day in one of the baby books, which made me giggle. It's true that baby poo can be a bit perplexing – and a common topic of conversation – when you're a new mum.
Nicola from Edinburgh, mum to Hannah, nine, and Feena, seven

I'd done a lot of research and I knew roughly what was normal and what wasn't, but I was still pretty shocked and disgusted by my first baby's nappies! It was weird the way her poo changed colour so many times.
Ellie from Poole, mum to Gina, twelve, Stewart, eight, and Julie, two

Those first nappies – it was like my baby was a tar machine! The more I tried to use cotton wool to dab it off the more it seemed to come out, and I ended up with it on my forehead, the bed sheets and the change bag. That first thick, black, newborn poop is something else!
Ruth from Newton Abbot, mum to Bethany, seventeen months, and Thomas, five months

I was lucky (depending on how you look at it) as I'd had an emergency C-section and my daughter did her first poo before I got out of bed, so my husband and mum had to change her. My hubby described it as like incredibly sticky Marmite!
Amanda from Fleet, mum to Tabitha, nine months

The first poo was like tar, thick and black, and it took ages to clean off. It then changed to a weird green colour before finally going yellow and becoming less thick.
Rachel from Staines, mum to Jake, five, Kyla, four, and Abigail, five months

My husband changed both the first nappies – in my first daughter's case, she missed the nappy and got his trousers instead! I was worried about the green poo in between the tar-like stuff and the yellow stuff – I'd heard somewhere it was a sign of bad colic so got into a right panic about it, only to be told by my health visitor that it was normal. But give me the thick stuff any day. It's no fun having to remove clothes because bright yellow runny poo has leaked on to them!
Clair from Portsmouth, mum to Chloe, two, and Megan, four months

Joey's first poo ended up all over him, me, my hospital gown and his towel! I don't even remember cleaning us up; the midwife and my husband must have taken care of it. I remember being worried about it getting into my perineal stitches, though. He was always prolific with his poos, at least one or two a day of that runny, seedy breastfed baby poo. He also went through a phase of doing very frothy, green poos, but despite a phone call to La Leche League, a visit to the health visitor, and excluding dairy from my diet for a fortnight, we never did get to the bottom of the matter (if you'll pardon the pun!), and it eventually went back to normal. He's now a lively, healthy lad and he still has good bowel habits!
Anna from Birmingham, mum to Joey, three

My first daughter had black, tar-like poo for a good three days or so – a very nice introduction to being parents! It's the most awful stuff to scrape off. My second daughter didn't have a poo at all until the 'limit' given by my health visitor was nearly up – about forty-eight hours, I think. But then it was more like a small, solid white plug, with just a little bit of black. Then it quickly became the usual mustard-seedy stuff. I actually quite like the smell of breastfed newborn poo as it's quite sweet and milky. Much better than the formula-fed or weaned variety!
Charlotte from Morpeth, mum to Leah, three, and Rebekah, nineteen months

6 Will she always have a birthmark?

Birthmarks are coloured marks that develop on or just below the skin, before or soon after birth. In most cases, the cause is unclear. They're very common, with as many as one in three babies born with one sort or another, and come in many different forms, ranging from very mild and superficial, to seriously disfiguring or even risky to health. Often, birthmarks will disappear or fade over time. However, some are permanent unless removed, and if your baby's appearance is badly affected, or there's a risk to her health, she may be offered treatment such as medication or laser surgery. Do talk to your GP if you're worried about a birthmark, as early diagnosis can be crucial.

If your baby's birthmark is disfiguring, it can come as a shock, and you may find it hard dealing with stares and comments. Give it time, if that's the case. Most parents find that a visible birthmark eventually becomes a unique feature that's very much part of their baby.

What the experts say

Dr David says: Most birthmarks – medically known as naevi – are harmless but some may require treatment for cosmetic reasons, or for a variety of medical ones. Very common, purely superficial birthmarks include salmon patches or 'stork bites', which are pink, flat and usually fade to nothing within a few years or even months; and Mongolian blue spots – dark areas of skin usually found on the bottom or back that are common in babies of African or Asian origin. These also tend to fade within four or five years. Café au lait spots are light brown patches which in most cases are completely harmless but if numerous, will need checking out as they can indicate a very rare but serious condition called neurofibromatosis.

A common form of birthmark is the haemangioma, often known as a strawberry mark because of its appearance, which is thought to affect about one in every ten babies. It's a collection of small blood vessels that form a lump under the skin, and will usually begin to appear and grow within a few days or weeks after birth. Strawberry marks may be either deep or superficial, and can appear anywhere on the body and sometimes internally, in which case doctors will probably want to carry out a scan to see if organs such as the liver are being affected. Special treatment is also likely to be necessary if a haemangioma develops near the eye, as it can have long-term effects on a child's vision; if one grows on the jaw, chin or neck, where it may affect the airways and lead to breathing difficulties; or if a haemangioma becomes ulcerated and infected. Depending on the size and location, treatment could involve medication in the form of antibiotics or steroids, laser treatment or surgery. However, the majority of haemangiomas don't cause a problem and will disappear on their own by the time a child is six or seven.

Port wine stains are also caused by an abnormal collection of blood vessels, which cause flat red, dark pink or purple marks on the skin, most commonly on the face although they can occur anywhere on the body. These will persist through childhood and tend to darken and thicken in adulthood. Although painless, they're permanent unless treated and may well have a psychological impact if they're visible. Often it's better to tackle them early, and as there are also a couple of very rare syndromes that are associated with port wine stains, it's a good idea to seek medical advice as soon as possible if your baby has one.

Crissy says: If your baby has a prominent birthmark it can bring forth a wide range of emotional responses. Having ruled out any significant health implications and explored all possible options, some mums feel sufficiently reassured to be able to take things in their stride. For others, the realisation that their baby looks 'different' can be traumatic and may leave them struggling to bond and feeling sad, guilty, anxious or angry. Being upset because your baby has a conspicuous birthmark doesn't make you a bad mother. It just makes you human. All mums naturally want what's best for their babies and so it's OK to grieve when things don't turn out as you hoped. Whatever your experience, it's important to give yourself some time to make sense of what's happening for you and your baby.

Once the initial shock has passed, most parents do find ways to come to terms with their baby's birthmark. Unfortunately, Western society attaches a substantial premium to our physical appearance and a visible birthmark will inevitably make your baby more noticeable. It's likely that some people will stare and may ask questions or make inappropriate, rude or upsetting comments. There's no reason why parents should feel obliged to put up and shut up when faced with such insensitive behaviour. It's fine to respond to hurtful comments, perhaps to ask someone not to stare or to offer a brief explanation, but emotions tend to run high when it comes to our kids, so always aim to be calmly assertive and try and avoid being drawn into a full-blown confrontation.

You may also encounter difficulties closer to home if friends or family members feel uncomfortable or unsure of whether to broach the subject of your baby's birthmark. If you strive to be open and upfront about matters the atmosphere will tend to be more relaxed for all concerned. As she grows your child will learn how to deal with having a distinctive birthmark by following the example you set. In showing unconditional acceptance and positive regard you are teaching your child that her birthmark is simply a feature she was born with, like her brown hair or blue eyes, and as such it does not make her somehow less than others or define who she is.

What the netmums say

Marked out

When my son was born he had a Mongolian blue spot that covered the top of his bottom and half of his back. I was told it would disappear by the time he was eighteen months old, but you can still see it faintly now. It didn't bother me at all, although there were occasions while getting him changed in public when I wondered if other mums would think it was bruising. Apparently, I had one when I was a baby, too.

Lucy from Oswaldtwistle, mum to Charlie, three

My daughter had eighteen haemangiomas on different parts of her body, which developed shortly after her birth. She's had many scans to make sure she didn't have any internally – which could have been dangerous – and luckily they were always clear. Some were just small dots and have since faded completely. However, the one on her cheek was aggressive, in spite of steroid injections to try and stop the growth, and became badly infected. Eventually it was so bad that they operated to remove it, as well as one on her head and one on her neck. She was eight months old at the time, and she had a further op to correct the scar at two. The one on her cheek is now very light, and we're very glad she had the surgery.

Sharon from Glasgow, mum to Jamie, seven, and Ewan and Anna, three

Joseph has a strawberry mark on his back which the doctor says is fine, but it's quite raised and I worry about catching it with my nail when getting him out of the bath or getting him dressed. He also has 'stork bite' marks on the bridge of his nose, on the back of his head and on the back of his neck just below the hairline. I'm not worried too much about these but I do hope the one on the bridge of his nose fades as it makes him look like he's always cross!

Laura from Aldershot, mum to Joseph, four months

My son developed a strawberry birthmark on his side shortly after birth. I was told it was nothing to worry about and it didn't bother or irritate him. It disappeared like they said it would, about eighteen months later.

Emma from Okehampton, mum to Owen, three

Morgan had a Mongolian blue spot on his bottom and most of his back, which remains there now though we've been told it will fade over time. When he was born the midwife pointed it out immediately and we were worried as we had no idea what they were then. It would have been helpful to know during pregnancy. Apparently they're extremely common among black and mixed-race babies.

Michelle from Birmingham, mum to Tyler, four, and Morgan, eleven months

My daughter developed a strawberry birthmark at about six weeks in the middle of her forehead and my health visitor assumed we'd hurt her and referred us to social services! It was a very difficult time. Since then I've lost count of the number of strangers and professionals who have queried it. She's two now and it's finally beginning to fade. My plea is, look and think before you comment about a child and a mark.

Karen from Liverpool, mum to Anna, two

I wasn't bothered in the slightest by Poppy's birthmark, which is a round, dark brown mark on her cheek, about 2 cm long and 1 cm wide. Yet people were wary and seemed uncomfortable mentioning it, in case it upset me. Even now, all I see is her cute, pretty face. I always tell her she's special and beautiful, and she's very positive about it. I'd never encourage her to have it removed, certainly not so young, but if she's unhappy in her teens and wants to look into the possibility, I'll support her.

Sara from Holt, mum to Poppy, four

Amber was born with a bright red birth naevus on her left wrist, about two inches across. It's not raised at all, and she pays it no attention. We've been told that it's nothing to worry about and will fade completely by the time she's six or seven – in fact, it's actually faded quite a lot already. The only concern, we've been told, is if she cuts or grazes it, and then we can expect it to bleed quite a lot.

Helen from Bexleyheath, mum to Amber, two

My little one has an extensive strawberry birthmark on her left cheek. It was there at birth, although only a faint outline, and within two weeks it began to swell. By eight weeks, it was ulcerated. Most people assume they're harmless but in her case, scans revealed it was growing behind her eye and near the brain. I found it so hard to cope with. Every time I looked at her all I saw was this huge birthmark and if I took her out, I'd lay her on that side in the pram so no one could see. I rejected her totally and feel very sad looking back. It's improved loads since she began a new treatment. I've even started worrying about how I'll feel when it's gone. I never thought I'd feel like that, but I've accepted that it's part of her.

Trudie from Billericay, mum to Josie, fourteen months

I have twin boys and my eldest has a birthmark on his face. It wasn't there when he was born and I can't remember when it did appear. It's on his right cheek and goes across his eye and up to his forehead. Thankfully it doesn't affect his eyes significantly, although the vision in his right eye isn't as good as in his left eye. He's halfway through a programme of laser treatment at the moment. We decided to have it done now, before he starts school. Kids can be cruel, and we didn't want him to be known as the twin with the birthmark.

Sarah from Woodford Green, mum to Joseph and James, two

7 Why is he squinting?

You'll no doubt be gazing into your baby's eyes quite a lot as you get to know him in the early weeks of his life. Sometimes, however, his eyes may appear to be looking in different directions, and you might wonder why.

There are two good reasons why babies squint – or at least, appear to be squinting – in their first few months, and neither are a cause for worry. If it's still a problem beyond that, though, it's important to flag it up with a health professional.

What the experts say

Louise says: Lots of newborns will appear to have a squint – the medical term is strabismus. During the first few months, the muscles round the eyes are still developing, which means they won't always be aligned – in fact, they can be all over the place! However, do mention it to your health visitor or GP if your baby has a squint that persists beyond four or five months – particularly if there's a family history of squinting – as true squints can be very damaging to eyesight and are best tackled early on.

Quite often, what appears to be a squint turns out to be what's known as a pseudo squint – it's an illusion, really, which occurs because babies often have a very flat bridge at the top of the nose. A pseudo squint will disappear as he gets a bit older, and his nose develops. But if there's any doubt about a squint, an eye specialist can carry out a quick, painless test to determine whether there's a problem or not.

What the netmums say

Babies who squint

As a first-time mum, I remember being worried that my son's eyes would occasionally go in different directions, but then I learnt after asking the HV that it takes a few weeks for newborns to be able to focus and control both eyes together. So as with so many things, it turned out to be nothing to worry about!
Lara from Northampton, mum to Trent, sixteen months

My son used to go cross-eyed sometimes up until he was about three months old, and I would wonder if he was all right, perhaps even partially sighted. My hubby was so worried about it for a while that he thought he might have brain damage. My health visitor was lovely and said that it was probably just due to under-developed eye muscles, and something to keep an eye on (so to speak). Thankfully, he gained more control over it as he got older – and his sight is fine. ·
Jessica from Bristol, mum to Marley, two

The double squint that my son has was at first put down to the bridge of his nose being wide. I was annoyed, because we've now been informed that if the health visitor had mentioned a squint earlier, it could have been solved with Botox instead of surgery. As it is a double squint, he can't have an eye patch either. Hopefully he will have the surgery before he starts school, as I worry that other children will bully him for it.
Laura from Carlisle, mum to Henry, twenty-one months

Our doctor told us at the six-week check that our son had a squint. Another doctor agreed, and we were referred to the eye hospital. We waited a long time for an appointment and when it finally

came he had a number of checks. But thankfully they said he had no evidence of a squint at all. He was fine.
Jenny from Bristol, mum to Tilly, five, and Finn, three

I've been keeping an eye on my daughter's eyes as the left one does have a slight turn. My sister had quite a bad squint when she was younger and had to have about eight different operations to correct it, so I'm well aware of the problems they can cause. I mentioned it to the health visitor at Grace's eight-to-twelve-month review. She's now got a referral to the eye clinic.
Katie from Bristol, mum to Grace, nine months

8 When will her cord stump drop off?

The shrivelled remains of your newborn's umbilical cord will be left sticking out from her tummy after your midwife clamps and cuts it at birth. This cord stump will usually hang around for a week or so before turning black and dropping off of its own accord, and the area should heal up completely soon afterwards. Some care is required in the meantime, as cord stumps can become sore and, occasionally, infected. Keep a close eye and chat to your midwife or health visitor if in doubt.

Once the healing's complete, your baby should be left with a scar in the form of a cute little belly button – although whether it's an 'innie' or an 'outie', there's no predicting. You may or may not wish to keep the cord clip, or even the stump itself, as a souvenir!

What the experts say

Louise says: Cord stumps will usually fall off within a week or so, with the area then taking a further week to ten days to heal, but sometimes the process can take up to three weeks. It's important to wait for it to drop off naturally – don't be tempted to pull it – and a good idea to try and fold down her nappy at the front to stop it catching or rubbing.

Meanwhile, aim to keep the stump and surrounding area clean and dry to help prevent infection. It's fine to submerge it so don't be put off bathing your baby if you want to. (For more on baths, see Question 12.) Water alone will be fine: you shouldn't need any kind of soap or cleanser. If you're topping and tailing, just gently wipe round the area with a little cotton wool and cooled, boiled water. Dry it gently by patting it with a towel before dressing her.

It will probably look a bit manky until it heals up. You may well notice a bit of clear fluid weeping around the area and that's nothing to worry about: in fact it's a sign that it's healing. As for smells, it will often be a bit pongy. However, if the smell's truly offensive, or if there are other indications such as fever or it's hot to touch or very red and swollen, it may be infected. Ask your health visitor or doctor to check if you're at all unsure.

Dr David says: It's not common, but if an umbilical stump does become infected it's important to get it treated, as the infection could in theory enter the body and that could cause a serious problem. A smelly discharge is usual and not in itself a problem, but my advice would be to get it checked out if your baby also has a temperature or seems ill in any other way, or if the skin around the belly button looks red and sore.

Occasionally a 'granuloma' can develop when inflammation at the base of the stump prevents normal skin tissue from developing – the area will remain red and unhealed and a persistent discharge may develop. Your GP, a practice nurse, or health visitor can cauterise the area with a chemical compound called silver nitrate – it's a simple procedure that is nothing to worry about. Meanwhile, keep a careful eye on the area in case infection develops and alert a health professional if you're worried.

What the netmums say

All about cord stumps

My fifth child's stump was horrendous – it absolutely stank of rotten eggs and was so bad you could smell it through her clothes. The health visitor said it was normal for some babies and was nothing to worry about. Luckily it only lasted two or three days then it fell off! *Nicola from Dewsbury, mum to Alice, sixteen, Mollie, thirteen, Harvey, eight, Matilda, four, and Kittie Flo, sixteen months*

Samuel's cord fell off at around ten days, straight into a nappy of poo. As I wanted to keep the clip as a souvenir, I put my hand in to retrieve it. I washed it under the tap and it's still in his baby book now.

Donna from Wolverhampton, mum to Samuel, five

On day four after the birth we had a check-up with the midwife, just to see how he was doing. She mentioned Jack's stump was rather smelly (it really was smelly, I've never smelt anything so bad in my life!) and that I should take him to the doctor that day. She said it didn't look red and sore but it was just the smell concerning her. I made an appointment for the following day but by then it had fallen off, looked fine, and no longer smelled!

Lisa from London, mum to Jack, four months

Saffia's stump fell off on day three and the area became smelly and gunky. I showed it to my midwife and she told me it was infected and that I should get it treated that day otherwise it could be fatal! I rang the GP in a panic only to be told that my midwife was overreacting. We were given an antibiotic cream and within a few days it had cleared up.

Jenna from Spalding, mum to Amber, three, and Saffia, twenty-one months

I was very cross that they clamped my son's cord in such a way it was pulling at his stomach. He was uncomfortable and would cry out if I held him front to front with me because he could not take the pressure on his cord. The midwife said they would not remove it before twenty-four hours was up, as it was not their policy. But I then spoke to a helpful, different midwife who led me through removing the clamp, with the aid of a pair of bolt cutters. I think it's worth warning parents that they should never try to prise the clamp apart or try to take it off without professional guidance, as it could cause a good deal of damage. My GP later told me that he saw a lot of babies who'd had their clamps removed improperly by parents.

Taliah from Worcester, mum to Kaydence, six, Aurelia, four, Nymeria, two, and Octavian, ten months

Connor's stump cord was fairly neat and I didn't have any problems keeping it clean. I'm a little squeamish and I'm glad it came
off inside his sleep suit. And yes, I have kept it for posterity!
Clare from Doncaster, mum to Connor, eighteen months

My first kept his stump for about four or five weeks, which was quite
a long time, and it did become a bit pongy. Whilst looking online
for advice about it I read some scary stuff about infected stumps,
but in fact there were no problems at all in the end. There was
lots of cheering when it finally fell off, we spent ages looking for it
and finally found it in the toe of his sleep suit! My second son lost
his at a more normal time – about ten days or so.
Hilary from Cardiff, mum to Samuel, two, and Edward, ten months

Joseph's cord fell off after four or five days. It was stinking by then,
so much that some non-parent friends thought he'd pooed! He
got a bit of an infection after it fell off but it cleared up within a
couple of days after the doctor gave us some cream. I knew about
cord care but didn't know that after it fell off his belly button would
be quite so sticky.
Laura from Aldershot, mum to Joseph, four months

I felt a little bit sad when the cord stump dropped off. It was the
last reminder that my babies had been attached to me inside my
belly.
Irma from Oldham, mum to Damir, four, and Aydin, two

9 Will his eyes and hair change?

Lots of parents want to know if, how and when their baby's appearance is likely to change – with particular interest in the ultimate colour of the eyes, or the type of hair that will replace those baby-soft locks. How these things pan out is down to your baby's unique genetic make-up – and genetics is a complex science, which means that whilst he *might* take after one or both of you in appearance, he might take after someone from an earlier generation, or he might just be his own little person. Quite possibly there'll be a mixture of influences going on. Fact is, his eyes and hair *are* very likely to change . . . but as to when and how, you will simply have to wait and see!

What the experts say

Louise says: Most white babies are born with eyes that are dark blue or slate grey, but as I'm often telling parents, they're very likely to change! That's because the pigment that gives eyes and skin its colour – known as melanin – doesn't develop until after birth, and it can be anything up to two or even three years before the ultimate colour is set. It's a change that can happen gradually – or virtually overnight. Black and Asian babies are *usually* born with brown or very dark, almost black eyes, which don't tend to change much. But there aren't really hard and fast rules – the bottom line is that eyes come in a huge range of hues. Often they'll be made up of more than one shade, and occasionally, one pair of eyes can be two different colours. You may well end up surprised by what your baby's turn out to be.

A mix of genes, pigmentation, and hormones mean that hair is also really variable, changeable – and unpredictable. Some babies are born with a whole head of hair, others are born bald. They will usually lose the hair they're born with, which tends to be soft and downy to start with, but it grows back a thicker texture, and very often a completely different colour. Early curls may grow back straight, or vice versa. But even then, it's still quite possible it will change some more in the years to come. Some parents wonder when their bald baby's hair will grow, and it can take a while. But there's not a lot that can be done about it – it's a myth that cutting it or brushing it will encourage growth. Bald spots are also very common, usually caused by your baby's sleeping or sitting in the same position.

There's not much point in trying to guess the way your baby's hair or eyes are going to turn out, because it's all down to a genetic lottery, really. Although my little girl ended up with my grey eyes, she's got very straight hair, in spite of the fact that her dad and I are both madly curly!

What the netmums say

All change?

Both my babies were born with loads of dark hair – everyone would comment on it. And they still have it, although Bethany had a bald spot on the back of her head from being laid flat in her cot. Her eyes were the first thing I noticed – huge and blue, with thick, dark eyelashes. I was warned they would probably change colour, but after seventeen months she still has the same bright blue shade she was born with. She's going to be a real heartbreaker!
Ruth from Newton Abbot, mum to Bethany, seventeen months, and Thomas, five months

All three of my children were born with tons of hair! Jake was born with a mass of dark, almost black, hair. This gradually lightened and it is now a light brown. Kyla was born with fluffy blonde hair. This fell out and she started to get really light ginger hair up until she was around thirteen months old and then it went bright blonde. Abigail was also born with fluffy blonde hair, which is now a light brown.

Rachel from Staines, mum to Jake, five, Kyla, four, and Abigail, five months

I don't actually remember when my daughter's eyes started changing. She was born with blue eyes and then at some point they started going brown and they're now very dark brown. It must have been a gradual thing.

Rose from Chesham, mum to Elsa, two

My eldest daughter was born with deep blue eyes but after a short while they changed to green and then at around three or four months old they eventually settled on a lovely chocolate brown. My youngest was born with eyes that were a deep blue and then became an array of colours – they went from blue to blue/grey colour, then they changed to a green and are now hazel. Her hair also changed colour: she was born with a darker mouse brown colour and as she got older her hair got lighter and it is now a lovely blonde. I was surprised because I assumed hair always went darker, not lighter. It's amazing how much they can change.

Hannah from Bolton, mum to Lucy, six, and Jessica, fifteen months

My son was born with bright red hair and we thought it was strange as both his dad and I have dark hair. However, afterwards it changed to white blonde and at two, he's still very fair. Who knows what colour it will end up eventually!

Emma from Stoke, mum to Jordan, two

My children are mixed race and their hair has changed loads since birth. My eldest had just a little bit of straight, mousy brown hair at the start, but it became more of a chestnut brown and, at ten months, went curly. The youngest came out with a headful of jet-black hair that was thick and glossy from day one. Her hair turned curly when she got to three months and hasn't stopped growing since.

Jane from Birmingham, mum to Casey, two, and Leanne, fourteen months

Connor was born with quite dark hair that slowly disappeared to be replaced with extremely blonde locks. His eyes were a deep blue, very wide with long lashes. At around four days old they looked like they were changing to a greeny-brown, but then at seven days they went back to dark blue.

Clare from Doncaster, mum to Connor, eighteen months

I was under the misapprehension that eye colour always followed Dad's so was surprised when mine were both born with grey eyes (their daddy's are brown) and they've stayed that way. It's a beautiful colour – but I may be biased!

Anna from Maidstone, mum to Dan, seven, and Lola, three

My daughter has never had very much hair and still doesn't have enough for it to be in any shape to be able to put a clip in it. Mind you, I was the same – my mum was convinced I'd be starting school without hair, so I don't hold out much hope of her growing some any time soon!

Lisa from Great Dunmow, mum to Luciana, nineteen months

Megan's always had hair but it was wispy when she was born, and more straight than curly. It's now incredibly curly, and on a bad day she looks like she has had a shock. There's nothing that will tame it!

Lindsay from Ballynahinch, mum to Megan, two

10 Shouldn't I love her more?

If you looked down into your baby's eyes after giving birth to her but didn't feel the lightning bolt of love you were expecting, you're not alone. Bonding is an important process, but it's by no means automatic after the birth and it may yet take a while before mother love consumes you. This is particularly so if you had a difficult birth, or if you've already got emotional difficulties on your plate, anyway.

Although it's extremely common to feel indifferent to your baby at first, an ongoing failure to bond can be an indication of postnatal depression, so do talk to someone about it if you're experiencing this problem, and make sure you get any help that you need. (For more on PND, see Question 19.)

What the experts say

Crissy says: There's a common and often damaging misconception that an intense mutual bond between mum and baby always occurs spontaneously within moments of birth. It can happen. Babies are born with an innate capacity to bond with others and most will be ready and able to begin bonding right away, naturally responding to the smell, sound and touch of their mothers. And it's just as well, because babies need to bond with their primary caregiver – usually their mum – if they're going to survive and thrive. A strong and reliable bond supports their emotional, physical, intellectual and social development, and the nature and quality of this attachment plays a crucial role in creating a lasting template for their future relationships.

However, 'instant' bonding is not the norm. Usually it will only take place after an uncomplicated delivery, when the baby is in good health and wide awake, and the mum is given whatever support she needs to hold and feed her little one. Bonding may well be a more complex process if you've had a difficult or traumatic birth; there's something wrong with your baby; you've been unable to cuddle her straight away; or if you're simply feeling shocked, sore and exhausted and your hormones are still raging.

Mums may also bring their own personal difficulties to the new relationship – a stressful home environment or lifestyle, neglectful or abusive childhood experiences, illness, depression, anxiety or low self-esteem can all make it difficult for a mum to engage with her baby and to be emotionally available and present. But even without such difficulties, it's not uncommon for a woman to feel disappointed, overwhelmed and frustrated by the demands of motherhood or to feel resentful or indifferent towards her baby for a while. Sometimes it can take days, weeks or even months before experiencing the first stirrings of an emotional connection with your baby, but in most cases, given time, it *will* happen. It's rarely a 'lightning bolt' moment, though. Often, mums describe the process as emerging gradually from the day-to-day experience of caring for their baby, and becoming aware of their attachment deepening over time as they and their baby become better acquainted.

Bonding is a co-created, mutual process. Just as you're working hard to decipher the signals your baby transmits with every sound and movement she makes, so in turn your baby will be watching you every bit as keenly, paying close attention to your tone of voice, facial expressions, gestures and emotions. When you successfully interpret her demands and her needs are consistently met, your baby begins to learn that she can trust you to take care of her. But you're a mum, not a mind reader, and so you don't need to get it right every time. In order to establish a secure attachment you don't have to successfully meet all of your baby's needs, all of the time; neither do you need to be a stay-at-home mum or be available 24/7. What you do need to be is a 'good-enough' mum, able to identify and satisfy your baby's needs more often than not. Bonding shouldn't feel like a test to be passed or failed, so try not to beat yourself up when you don't always know how best to soothe your baby or if you sometimes struggle to offer her your undivided attention or unconditional love and affection. What will make it easier is if there's plenty of emotional and practical support on hand to bolster your confidence, take some of the pressure off and allow you to catch up on lost sleep and precious 'me' time.

But try, as well, to make sure that you get plenty of relaxed and leisurely time together with your baby – it'll be an essential investment in your relationship. Spend time cuddling, stroking and gently massaging your little one and, where possible, try to include some skin-to-skin time. You may feel like you're just going through the motions for a while yet, but wherever possible try to find a smile, keep your face animated and make eye contact with your baby. Talk to her, read her the paper, sing along with the radio and carry her round the supermarket in a sling rather than a pram. Worrying and feeling guilty that you haven't yet bonded just cranks up the pressure even higher, so try to be patient and compassionate with both yourself and your baby and in time, the rest will almost certainly follow.

What the netmums say

You can't hurry love

My initial feeling after both my children's births was . . . nothing! I didn't get that rush of love that everyone talks about; I was just numb and flat. I knew I loved them and would care for them, but there was no tidal wave of emotion. Over the first few weeks, as the bond deepened, I started to chill out and enjoy things more. Having spoken about it with friends since, it seems most of them didn't feel a whoosh of love, either.
Yvonne from Ayr, mum to Damien, four, and Quinn, two

With both my wonderful girls, I wouldn't say I bonded straight away. It was a nurturing love at first sight but I think, with both, I only

bonded with them after four or five months when I felt their person-
alities starting to develop and I could interact with them. Since then
our bonds have grown, and I believe will continue to evolve and
become stronger. I think as mums we develop our relationships with
our children in the same way that we develop all our emotional
feelings. For some it's instant, for some it grows, and for some it
takes work and possibly help. Hopefully, we all get there in the end.
*Emma from Worcester Park, mum to Niamh, three, and Fionnuala,
eight months*

My little one was born by emergency C-section, and my partner
was the first one to hold her, feed her, and help change her bum.
I was very groggy and shaky after the section, so I got my skin-to-
skin contact with her but wasn't really allowed to do much with
her at first, and I don't think I bonded with her straight away. It
took a few days, once I was able and allowed to do things for
her myself. Now I adore her.
Natalie from Rossendale, mum to Niobe Grace, one month

Rhys was born via forceps after a normal pregnancy and quick
labour. I think I found it all quite surreal and couldn't get my
head round the fact that he was finally here. It therefore took
me a while to develop a bond. I remember vividly the moment
I fell in love with him though. He was three weeks old. I felt a
rush of love that filled me with the best feeling in the world – so
strong it ached. It's amazing.
Holly from Poole, mum to Rhys, six months

I had complications, and an emergency C-section, and was in
hospital for ten days. I couldn't walk properly or even pick my son
up. My husband had to do everything for a while and to this day
Adam is a 'daddy's boy'. Rightly or wrongly, I reckon that's to do
with the events following his birth. I can't really say when the bond
happened. To be honest, it took months. He was not an easy baby
and I had no confidence. But then I started feeling defensive when
people tried to advise me on bringing him up. I felt myself putting
an invisible arm around him, and thinking, 'Shut up, this is my son,
I'll do things my way!' I knew then I did love him. My heart was

pounding with the protective love only a mum can feel.
Sally from Corby, mum to Adam, three

When my son was born, I looked at him not quite believing he was mine and to be honest, not really feeling anything, except guilt that I wasn't feeling anything! I struggled for eleven days to feed and spent most of that time praying he would sleep just a bit longer than an hour and a half at a time, to give my poor breasts a break. I eventually gave up trying on day twelve, gave him a bottle and he slept for four hours. I clearly remember, two weeks after he was born and I'd been able to get some sleep, looking at him asleep on the bed and feeling such an overwhelming, all-consuming rush of utter love, I actually cried. I've never looked back.
Lindsey from Wirral, mum to Sam, two

I didn't bond with my first two children. I suffered both antenatal and postnatal depression with both, which wasn't detected for a long time. It only really hit me when they were three and two. One day I woke up and it dawned on me that I actually loved them. It was overwhelming. My third was born by emergency C-section under a general anaesthetic. I didn't bond instantly, but I got that overwhelming love when he was around six weeks. I now love all my children unconditionally and feel guilty that it took so long with my first two.
Hayley from Manchester, mum to Ellie, five, Harrison, four, and Jacob, three months

I thought I would bond with my daughter instantly and felt like a failure when I didn't. It wasn't until she was twelve weeks that my instincts kicked in and I realised just how crazy I was about her. I hadn't realised it's normal not to bond instantly, hence the reason I felt like a bad mum. When I had my son two years later I was besotted from the minute I saw him. I just couldn't stop looking at him or cuddling him. I think I was overcompensating for how guilty I felt about my daughter. It's the one piece of advice I would give to any expectant mum: don't feel bad if the bonding doesn't happen straight away. I wish I'd been told that myself.
Eleanor from Wishaw, mum to Kaity, four, and Adam, two

With my first child I definitely did not bond immediately. In fact, at five months I confessed to my husband that I did not feel like he was mine, I felt more like his childminder. Despite breastfeeding and caring for him, it felt as though his real mummy was going to arrive at any minute to take him away. I'd been convinced the whole pregnancy that the baby was a girl, and was truly shocked to find it was a boy. At that time I felt like all my maternal instinct was gone. Once he was around seven months old, I started to feel like I would perhaps be upset if another woman did come and take him away. I think that was the start of feeling bonded. Gradually, I began to notice there were things about this baby that I enjoyed. It was a slow process – definitely not love at first sight. With my subsequent children there was more of a bond from the start, an instant knowledge that I had a deep unconditional love for them.

Kate from Folkestone, mum to Luke, six, Mia, four, and Thomas, two

Sadly, I didn't bond immediately. I had a stressful labour followed by an emergency C-section and it took me a while to come around. When I first saw my little girl she was fast asleep and it didn't quite feel real. It was almost like she wasn't mine. She then spent the next four days screaming every night while I struggled with breastfeeding, which I found very stressful and painful. So the bond between us was gradual. She's eight months now, and I seem to love her more and more every day.

Kim from Ipswich, mum to Jessica, eight months

PART TWO: 0–3 MONTHS

11 Is breastfeeding supposed to be this difficult?

If you've run into problems with breastfeeding, you're not alone. For some mums it becomes hard going – perhaps because it's more painful, exhausting, or restrictive than they had imagined, because of difficulties getting a baby to feed or anxiety about milk flow, or because of a specific problem such as mastitis or thrush. Mums who do carry on through difficulties early on in breastfeeding tend to agree it clicks into place after the first month or two. So, if you've hit a rough patch but you're determined to feed your baby for the optimum six months that's officially recommended, or beyond, then your best bet is to seek as much help as you can in finding a solution, and battle on.

If, on the other hand, difficulties with breastfeeding are making you truly miserable; are causing problems for other members of the family; or are prompting genuine concern about your baby's health or growth, then you should certainly consider the alternatives. For some mums, it can be disappointing having to ditch or reduce breastfeeds – for others, a relief. Either way, it's not something you need to feel guilty about. As long as your baby's getting the nourishment he needs to thrive, he'll be doing fine.

What the experts say

Maggie says: Pain is often cited as a reason why mums struggle with breastfeeding. Some soreness is quite normal in the early weeks, but if it's severe, or prolonged, or your nipples are actually cracked or bleeding, it's probable your baby isn't latched on properly. Ask your health visitor or a breastfeeding counsellor to check that you're doing it right. In the meantime, nipple shields may help, although they have disadvantages because they can be off-putting for a baby and you lose out on skin-to-skin contact. And lots of mums swear by cabbage leaves, cooled in the fridge and then placed in the bra – there's no medical evidence in their favour, but they do seem to provide relief! If you want to try a nipple cream, I tend to recommend Lansinoh, which contains an ingredient called highly purified anhydrous lanolin (HPA). It's good for both prevention and healing as it provides a breathable barrier, keeps skin moist, and helps to protect against mastitis. And as it's organic, it doesn't need to be wiped away before feeding.

Although comfort sucking can be a good thing, because it helps stimulate milk production and is a good way to bond, and for mum to get a rest, it might be wise to try limiting it if your breasts are sore. Most babies tend to take what they need in the way of milk within about ten to twenty minutes or so, but you can tell for sure if he's finished feeding by putting your little finger in his mouth and gauging the strength of his suck. It won't be as strong if he's only looking for comfort.

Do ask for help from your health visitor or GP if you really are in pain. You could be suffering from mastitis – a painful inflammation of the breast that can become infectious and cause flu-like symptoms – or from thrush, a fungal infection that often develops in a baby's mouth and is then passed on to his mum. You can get safe treatments to clear these problems up and meanwhile you should try to continue feeding if you don't want your milk supplies to be affected. If you're diagnosed with mastitis, massaging the affected area can also help.

In most cases, with the right help, breastfeeding problems can be overcome. But sometimes, it's just not in the interests of either mum, baby, or the wider family to keep going when the problems are severe or they're causing unhappiness. As a health visitor I absolutely support breastfeeding, but not at the expense of what's best for those involved. And bottle-feeding with love (as well as scrupulous attention to hygiene, and to making up feeds as directed) is just as good. (For more on sterilising bottles, see Question 22.)

Louise says: Anxiety over milk production is a common story, and sadly, it often leads to breastfeeding mums giving up before they really wanted to. The fact is that pretty much all mums will be able to produce enough milk for their baby, regardless of boob size. Usually when there doesn't seem to be enough milk it's to do with supply and demand – the less the baby suckles, the less milk is produced. And often, mums worried they're not giving their babies enough may offer a bottle as a supplement, with the result that milk supply *is* reduced. If you're concerned, try to feed your baby as frequently as possible. (For more on milk supply concerns, see Question 14.) Lots of mums lose track of feeds, so keeping a diary is a good idea. Skin-to-skin contact is a good way to get milk flowing, so one of the best things you can do if you're worried about your milk supply is to strip to the waist and just cuddle your baby to you – better still, get naked, get into bed with him and stay there, preferably for a whole day or more. (But be wary of falling asleep with him – for more on bedsharing, see Question 4.) Fenugreek is a natural remedy said to improve milk production – you can buy it in tablet form from health-food shops. There's no medical evidence it works, but many mums find it helps. I certainly did – although it's pungent stuff and it left me smelling pretty bad! In very special cases, a GP can prescribe medication to increase milk supply. But what's really important if you're worried about not having enough milk for your baby is getting help as soon as possible.

As far as sore breasts are concerned, I'm afraid it's often a question of perfecting your technique, and waiting for your nipples to 'wear in'. One natural remedy is to rub a little breast milk on them, as it has antiseptic properties. Keeping your boobs really clean and dry will also help, which is why it's important to use good-quality, really absorbent breast-pads, and to change them regularly.

If pain – for whatever reason – gets really bad, it might help to try changing your feeding position. Or you could express your milk and offer it to your baby in a bottle for a while. Often problems occur in just one breast – so perhaps you could express from the one for a while and continue feeding with the good one, until the problem gets sorted.

Whatever's causing breastfeeding difficulties, do seek help. I think it's a good idea to have a breastfeeding 'buddy', who's happy to offer moral support when you need it. Pick your buddy carefully, though – it needs to be someone neutral who can be relied on to make you feel better, not worse.

Of course, if you do come to a point where you want to stop breastfeeding, that's entirely your right. It's not just about what's best for your baby, it's about what's best for you and for your mental health. You may also need to take into account your partner's feelings and the needs of the rest of your family. Don't allow anyone to make you feel guilty for doing what you feel is right.

Dr David says: Something that occasionally causes problems for breastfeeding babies is a condition called tongue tie, or ankyloglossia, to give it the correct medical term. It occurs when an infant has a short frenulum – the piece of skin that joins the tongue to the floor of the mouth – which causes restriction of movement in the tongue. If you suspect it's a problem that's affecting your baby and preventing him from feeding properly, do ask your GP for advice. It can be treated with a simple surgical procedure.

Crissy says: Deciding whether to carry on through difficulties with breastfeeding, or to give up and reach for the formula is a difficult choice that many mums face. One of the biggest myths is that all women possess some intuitive knowledge and innate ability to feed their babies, but whilst the majority of women are physically capable of breastfeeding, in most cases, mum and baby need support and guidance to learn the skills that enjoyable and pain-free breastfeeding requires, and it's common for women to find breastfeeding a struggle at first. All too often, the level of support and advice offered in the early weeks of breastfeeding is not equal to the task, and a mum who feels unsupported, obligated or destined to fail is far more likely to turn to the formula than someone who feels adequately supported when the going gets tough.

You need to be compassionate and patient with yourself and your baby during this tricky learning period – after all, raging hormones, exhaustion and the aches and pains of early motherhood are already a recipe for meltdown. Allow yourself a few false starts, keep your goals realistic and achievable and remember that it's OK to need extra help and advice. If you can get the support you need to overcome any difficulties and persevere with breastfeeding, you're very likely to find it a deeply rewarding experience.

On the other hand, if you decide to drop breastfeeding, you should do so without regret. The 'breast is best' lobby is a powerful one so it's hardly surprising that those who choose not to, or feel unable to breastfeed, feel guilty. Somewhere along the way, whether or not a woman breastfeeds her baby seems to have become a measure of how good a mother she is. While for some women breastfeeding can be an empowering and life-enriching experience, for others the physical, emotional or social challenges can seem less of a dream and more of a nightmare. Not breast-feeding your baby for whatever reason should not invite misplaced and misinformed moral judgements – if you're getting grief from anyone about your choice, politely ignore them. At the end of the day, we all want what's best for our kids, and the best gift any baby can receive is a contented mum.

What the netmums say

A sore subject

Breastfeeding was a nightmare for me. Laila struggled to latch on and lost a lot of weight. We had to go back into hospital where they hooked me on to breast pumps, but very little came out. It would take Laila ages just to latch on, only for her to feed for a few minutes before falling asleep. It was very painful, and very depressing. I was scared to suggest bottle-feeding, as the midwives seemed dismissive of it. Finally, one suggested a combination of breast, expressing and formula, but it made me feel my whole life revolved around feeding! After six weeks, we went fully on to formula. She gained weight, slept well and got into a routine. And I stopped worrying. Finally I knew she was getting the food she needed.
Jenny from Stockport, mum to Laila, two

I had problems with both of mine and despite being determined to breastfeed I had to stop early with both of them. My son had tongue tie and I knew something wasn't right, but it wasn't diagnosed until he was seven weeks old. Although he had the tie snipped three times it regrew and eventually I gave up. I wonder now if my daughter had the same condition as she was the same – I stopped after two weeks with her and didn't feel anyone wanted to listen.

Tracy from Oldbury, mum to Alana, six, and Alfie, ten months

If at first you don't succeed, try, try again. Well, that's how I've bumbled through anyway. First time round I breastfed for a few months then got hospitalised with mastitis and found feeding from then on very stressful, so finally moved to formula. Jessica is certainly none the worse for it. This time round things are going well. Ethan seems to be able to empty a boob in less than five minutes and he's gaining weight rapidly and producing plenty of soiled nappies. Ultimately, you should do what's best for you and for the whole family. There's no point persisting with breastfeeding if everyone involved becomes frazzled.

Debbie from Croespenmaen, mum to Jessica, five, and Ethan, two months

I made a good start with breastfeeding but by day four I wasn't producing enough milk and – even though he was properly latching on – I had sore, bleeding, cracked nipples that were agony. So I swapped to bottles and formula. With an older child and a toddler too, it's been more practical for me to formula feed. I'm glad I gave it a shot, though.

Nicole from Bournemouth, mum to Toby, six, Anise, sixteen months, and Lukas, three months

Soon after his birth, my son was diagnosed with a cleft palate, which meant he was unable to feed from me. So for three months, I expressed every feed. However, I would not recommend it. New mums are so pressured. I felt so guilty at the thought of not providing him with my milk, I was a mess for weeks. And I was basically a milk cow: express for thirty minutes, feed for thirty minutes, wash up and sterilise everything, twenty minutes for a wee and a cuppa, then start all over again. My daughter was a dream on the breast. But she'd take almost nothing in the morning then 'power feed' for four hours later in the day. At six months, she got a snotty cold and decided bottles were easier. A happy, relaxed mum is more important than the method of milk delivery. If you need to stop breastfeeding due to pain/stress/sanity, then do.

Anna from Newton Abbot, mum to Isaac, three, and Milly, two

My daughter fed straight away and had no problems. However, I ended up with badly cut nipples and I found the pain so excruciating I would scream when she latched on. Fortunately my midwife, who's also a family friend, was a star. She helped me to try different positions and encouraged me not to give up – this support was absolutely key to my continuing. After three weeks the pain went, and I loved feeding time. Persevering through the pain was one of the hardest things I've ever done but I went on to breastfeed my little girl for fourteen months.

Claire from Chelmsford, mum to Ava, eighteen months

Jake was my first baby and I intended to breastfeed. Unfortunately, I wasn't shown how to feed him correctly and he didn't latch on right. I kept trying, but Jake kept screaming, so we gave him formula and he became a calm, contented baby. With Kyla, I was on anti-depressants and advised not to breastfeed at all. But with our third, Abigail, I decided to give it another shot. She took to it well, and this time round I wasn't afraid to ask for the help I needed. It was harder than I imagined, especially early on and during growth spurts when she wanted to feed a lot, but things got easier. I just needed to relax, and not get so worked up with worry about how much she was taking.

Rachel from Staines, mum to Jake, five, Kyla, four, and Abigail, five months

I had no problems feeding my daughter at hospital. She latched on no problem, got her fill, and fed routinely. The problems came at home. I was tender from the C-section I'd had, and trying to feed her in bed. I ended up with a sore back, cracked nipples, and a hungry baby. The midwife explained that I had the wrong positioning and Jemima wasn't latching on properly. I found a really comfortable padded chair, propped her up with the help

of a couple of pillows, and the problem disappeared. Never be too scared to ask for help.
Rachael from Accrington, mum to Jemima Katie, eight months

With both babies, I suffered excruciating nipple pain for the first few minutes of each feed, for several weeks. One midwife told me the pain meant I wasn't getting her latched on properly but I don't think that was true. I then caused myself more discomfort by unlatching (putting my finger down the side of her cheek to break the suction) and trying again, only to experience the same pain. Thankfully the whole process became easier after a while. Despite all the focus on breastfeeding, I don't think mums should be made to feel guilty if they choose not to. Personally I'm glad to do it for the ease and convenience. It's good for her, and it's helped me lose weight. But it's not for everybody.
Briony from London, mum to Mpilika, three, and Yenga, four months

With my first daughter, it took four days and a lot of tears from both me and her before the midwife realised I wasn't producing anything at all. I had milk for my second daughter, but she just refused point blank to latch on! I expressed for four weeks before my boobs dried up so she's now on formula. Both times I felt like a failure. But a fed baby is a happy baby.
Clair from Portsmouth, mum to Chloe, two, and Megan, four months

I had a lot of problems feeding my youngest. He had tongue tie and could not attach to my breast, but I only found this out when he was almost four months old. Feeding him was so stressful and I felt like a failure, as I'd never had problems feeding my eldest. I could not accept giving up and expressed every single feed for him. When the GP finally discovered what the problem was I decided to give up. My whole life revolved around expressing and I felt like a cow. Looking back, I wish I'd given him formula sooner.
Irma from Oldham, mum to Damir, four, and Aydin, two

After my milk came in, I was in excruciating pain at every feed for about six weeks. I just kept telling myself that it would get better, and it did. It helped that my partner was always there to stroke my back or my forehead, get me a drink and comfort me. As a result I'm still breastfeeding, six months on.

Alison from Halifax, mum to Imogen, six months

My nipples were left blistered by the first feed and after that, I really struggled and was very disheartened. It felt like a big disappointment when I finally gave in and gave him a bottle instead. Two weeks later, when there seemed less pressure, I tried offering the breast again and he latched on and started drinking. For a while I managed to feed him during the day, with a bottle at night. But at three months, for some reason, he stopped wanting any breast and I switched permanently to the bottle. I felt very un-needed. However, he's now a very healthy little man of ten months. I believe it doesn't matter whether your baby breastfeeds or bottle-feeds – as long as he feeds.

Anne-Marie from Royston, mum to Thomas, ten months

I found it so difficult! Jacob was struggling to latch on and I ended up with bleeding, engorged breasts and then mastitis. I have a Medela breast-pump so was able to express, which was still painful but much less so than breastfeeding. After two weeks of struggling, my mum, who's a midwife, bought me some nipple shields and they proved a lifesaver. I weaned him off them after two and a half months of use and we've been fine since then.

Natalie from Manchester, mum to Jacob, eleven months

12 How do I bath her?

Stripping an unwilling baby and submerging her in water is a baby-care basic that can leave the most confident of parents feeling nervous. 'How to bath your baby' demonstrations used to be part and parcel of a hospital stay after birth, but with maternity staff often pressed for time, and short stays now the norm, it's quite likely you'll be facing this particular learning curve without any instruction.

As with so much about looking after your newborn, giving her a bath is something that will become easy with time and experience – and chances are, it will eventually become a ritual that you both enjoy. In the meantime, practice makes perfect!

What the experts say

Maggie says: I remember shaking with fear when bathing my eldest for the first time – even though I'd worked on a maternity ward, and as a neo-natal intensive care nurse. So I know from experience that it's enough to leave any new parent in bits.

Many newborns don't like baths. They will often hate being stripped off and vulnerable, so it's a good idea to make bath time brief in the early days. In fact, you don't need to bath her at all initially, as you can do a perfectly good job of keeping her clean by 'topping and tailing' – in other words, washing all the bits that need washing with cotton wool and water. Use a clean bit of cotton wool for each area and attend to the eyes first, using cooled boiled water and wiping from the inside out to avoid the spread of infection. Make sure the room is warm and keep as much of her covered as possible while you're doing it.

When bathing your baby, you may have to use a process of trial and error to work out what feels best for you both. Baby baths can be problematic if you've had a C-section or have got a bad back – if you put them inside the big bath you've got to bend over, and if they're on the floor, or a stand or table, you've still got to lift them up to empty them. Help may be required. The kitchen sink is a perfectly good option while she's small enough, and saves the cost of any equipment – as long as your sink's nice and clean.

Whatever you do, make sure your baby's firmly and safely supported throughout. You can do this with one hand and arm, keeping the other free to wash her. There are also lots of good, age-appropriate devices on the market such as cradles or seats designed to keep baby safely in place and your hands free to wash her. Even with one of these, though, from a safety point of view it's crucial that you don't leave your baby for a second while she's in the bath, so make sure you've got everything you need close to hand before you start.

Lots of parents find the easiest thing is just to bring their baby into the bath with them. It can be lovely, but you really need another adult to help if you're going to do this because trying to climb in and out of the bath whilst holding a little one isn't a good idea from a safety point of view. You also need to be happy taking a bath in warm rather than hot water. The temperature of baby bath water should be comfortably warm but never hot and of course, you should always test it before putting her in.

Conventional wisdom has it that it's best to stick with plain water for newborns as their skin is so delicate, but recent research has found there may actually be some protective benefits in using a mild, gently cleansing baby bath product. Just make sure that whatever you use has been clinically tested and formulated specific-ally for infant skin. You should be able to get a good idea of what's suitable by checking the labels before you buy. But as a general rule, if any product seems to irritate or dry your baby's skin, stop using it and try something else – or switch to plain water, instead.

What the netmums say

Having a splashing time

Bathing was the only 'new mum' thing that terrified me! It was a while before I found the courage to do it for the first time – and even then I got my mum to come and help me. It was such a relief when I'd done it. I recommend the use of a baby bath thermometer, which I still use every day, as I have little sense of temperature. Also, a bath stand and a 'Cuddledry' hooded towel make things easier. I had no such fears with my second baby, I'm glad to say.
Camilla from Ipswich, mum to Savannah, two, and Willow, six months

William hated being bathed until he was about three months old, so for a while I'd call on my mum to do it most nights. I preferred to put him in the big bath rather than in the baby bath, so I'd take his car seat into the bathroom, and lay a towel over it. This gave me something safe to put him in for a few moments after taking him out. The only advice I could give is: don't panic, you're not going to drown your baby! I was so paranoid that something bad was going to happen that it wasn't until later that I realised how lovely bath time could be.
Marianne from Uddingston, mum to William, twenty-two months

Bathing twins is a challenge! My husband works as a chef, so he's not home for the bath and bed routine. In the early days, I had to leave one baby on the floor and bath them one at a time, getting each baby fully dressed afterwards. Bathing babies can be scary – they seem so small and fragile. I was always nervous about it, every time. It's easier now as they can sit up, so they get bathed together and they love it.
Cat from Edinburgh, mum to George, six, and Freyja and Tavia, eleven months

I was lucky in a way as we were in the special care baby unit for a while and the lovely nurse there taught me how to bath Isaac

before we left. It's scary when they are so tiny but both mine have always loved bath time, right from day one. They would float and relax in the water for as long as I would let them. Now my son's three, and his sister is two, and double bath time is so much fun I struggle to get them out!
Anna from Newton Abbot, mum to Isaac, three, and Milly, two

When my daughter was born, the nurse used her to demonstrate bathing, and ended up trying to say how much babies love baths over her screaming! My mum later told me the same thing happened when I was born, and I hated baths for years. So I made sure my sons' first baths were at home – and they liked it from the start. I found the baby bath too heavy to move or even just tip with water in it, so before long I was sitting in the bath with them while breastfeeding, which made it much easier. That's my tip: if all else fails, sit in the bath yourself with them. They were all fascinated to see my hair swish about in the water! I also found that it's best to feed either shortly before or during the bath – you might need a second adult to pass the baby to you or to take them from you – and to do it when they aren't tired.
Abi from Mitcham, mum to Alice, eight, Byron, five, and Phoenix, eight months

We bought one of those baby baths with arms that stretch over the top of your own bath, but my baby seemed so big and heavy to me, and I was scared I wouldn't be able to hold her upright for long enough to bathe her. My other half knew of my fears and decided to 'help' by taking what he thought was a clearly terrifying task off me and do it himself while I was resting one evening. But I was upset that this little landmark moment had been taken from me and my other half was horrified that I was so upset!
Catherine from Preston, mum to Megan, three

I've always used one of those plastic bath seats that hold the baby safely and leave your hands free to wash. I wouldn't be without it, as babies are so slippery.
Julie from Lichfield, mum to Eve, twelve, Charlie, two, and Amy, seven months

If I was on my own, I used a baby bath seat to strap her into so that I had both hands free to wash her, or if my husband was at home I had a bath with her and he would take her out and dry and dress her so I didn't have to climb out of the bath and hold her at the same time. My main concern was (and still is) her slipping from my grasp when lifting her out or passing her to my husband. She's always been one for being in deeper than usual water, she likes it up to her chest, keeping her warm, and she's always been a water baby, which makes it easier to wash her hair. She's quite happy to have jug of water tipped over her.
Sarah from Westgate-on-Sea, mum to Katie, eighteen months

I had a C-section so there was no bending for me. We had a table in the bedroom that we put her baby bath on. Make sure you have everything before bathing – I had a Post-it note on the door with a list of what I needed (that's baby brain for you!). I'd wrap her in a towel and cradle her in one arm to wash her hair then lay her in the water, and very gently hold her arm furthest from me so her neck had support from my arm. It seemed the most natural position for me. I only used a very little unperfumed baby wash so she wouldn't be too slippery, and then just splashed her all over with a baby sponge. Then she would be out and snugly wrapped up in a big towel! After drying her I'd give her a little massage before dressing her. I loved that time. Once I'd recovered from the section, we moved into the big bath with help from a baby bath support, which was great – I'd fold a muslin square on to it so she could lie on that rather than the plastic. With both hands free, I could enjoy a good play and splash with her.
Shirley from Bracknell, mum to Jessica, two

No one ever showed me how to bath a baby, so I just got on with it! I had a baby bath with a body support so I just needed to hold his head and make sure everything was ready, at arm's reach. So long as the temperature of the water was right and there was a towel ready to get him warm and wrapped up straight out the water, then we were all happy. My boys all loved baths from the start. I bathed them for the first time a week or two after birth, then

every other day until they started weaning and getting really grotty, and started needing one daily!
Ingrid from Warwick, mum to Jadon, three, Caleb, twenty-one months, and Bram, four months

The first time round I tried all different baby bathing equipment, but with my second child I didn't bother as I realised it was just as easy to do without. I didn't bath my second child until she was two and a half weeks old and I only bath her once a week. This makes my in-laws laugh, but at this age I don't think they need one more often.
Becky from Waterlooville, mum to Eleanor, four, and Hope, two months

My midwife showed me how to bath my baby in my kitchen sink as I didn't have a baby bath at that point. I then bought one that would fit in the kitchen sink so I could continue to bath her there for a while – no bending was required; there was no risk of the bath actually falling off the top; and no worries if the water splashed everywhere.
Emi from Sheerness, mum to Rosa, three

13 Is it OK to give him a dummy?

Dummies certainly seem to provoke strong feelings in parents – and a distinct sniff of disapproval from many health professionals. But while it's true that a pacifier as permanent accessory isn't a good look in a walking, talking toddler, and there are drawbacks associated with excessive dummy use, there's no doubt they can be useful for calming or comforting some babies – especially those that are particularly 'sucky', or those with colic (see Question 15).

As with lots of parenting tactics, the key seems to be moderation. Aim to restrict dummy use to sensible levels. And bear in mind that whilst some babies are happy to drop dummy habits without too much persuasion, or even of their own accord, some cling on determinedly. So one distinct advantage in *not* giving your baby one is that you'll never have to try taking it away. Don't be surprised, however, if your baby doesn't seem to want a dummy when offered: lots don't! (For more on ditching the dummy, see Question 46.)

What the experts say

Louise says: A dummy is a perfectly reasonable parental choice, as long as you moderate the frequency with which your baby has one. Think about why you're offering it, when you offer it for the first time. If it's a short-term technique for settling a baby who won't seem to settle any other way, then it could be a godsend. What you don't want to do is start a habit that will eventually mean he's sucking the dummy more often than not. Aim to offer it just when he needs settling or comforting, and keep it tucked away at all other times.

If you're breastfeeding, it's a good idea not to introduce a dummy for four to six weeks, while he's still getting feeding sussed. That's because sucking on a dummy requires a different technique to sucking on a nipple, and it's possible your baby will get confused and distracted by the dummy, to the detriment of feeding – it's known as 'nipple confusion'.

Health visitors tend to recommend you get rid of the dummy altogether before your baby turns one, and it makes sense. That way, you know you're not going to risk any potential problems with his speech and language development or with misalignment of teeth. These problems are only really linked to severe pacifier habits, so carefully restricted dummy use that goes even beyond that period is unlikely to be a problem. However, most parents find it's easier to get shot of a dummy sooner rather than later, when the habit is even more entrenched.

If your baby has a dummy, you do have to pay careful attention to hygiene, because they can harbour bacteria and that means an increased risk of ear or tummy infections. Sterilise dummies daily, and have a good collection so you've always got a clean one to hand. If you're likely to need one whilst out and about, make sure you also take a spare in a sterilised pot. Throw dummies away immediately if they become damaged, as bacteria can hide in the cracks. And never suck your baby's dummy to clean it. Our mouths are full of germs!

Maggie says: I'm not against dummies at all. If you've got a very sucky baby and a dummy is the only way you can get him to settle, then dummies are a good idea. But there are pros and cons to consider, and I'd recommend getting rid of it before your baby's first birthday and preferably from about six months of age, since it's easier to take them away the younger they are. Speech and language therapists caution against their use as it's felt they can impair speech development – a baby sucking on a dummy is less likely to engage, vocalise, babble and copy facial expressions and mouth movements. They're not popular with dentists either, as excessive use can cause misalignment of teeth and, where parents are tempted to dip dummies in something sweet – which is a very bad idea – dental caries. On top of that, dummy use is associated with an increased risk of gastrointestinal infections, oral thrush and earache.

One of the main drawbacks is that if your baby needs one to settle to sleep, a dummy becomes an unhelpful sleep association – in other words, he will only be able to get to sleep once he's sucking on his dummy, and so you're very likely to be getting up in the night to replace it if it drops out of his mouth. You could be making the proverbial rod for your own back by offering one in the first place! From that point of view, you're better off if he can suck his own thumb, fingers or fist – although the counter-argument to that is that thumb-sucking is even more likely to cause dental problems, because you can't take a thumb away, and therefore it's a habit that may be carried on well into childhood.

Current advice from the Foundation for the Study of Infant Death (FSID) is that giving a baby a dummy when putting him down to sleep can reduce the risk of cot death. The reasons for this are unclear, but it's thought a dummy can prevent a baby sleeping too deeply. However, they do also advise that you should wait for a month after birth, or until breastfeeding is well established, before offering a dummy, and that you aim to wean him off it after six months and before he's a year old. You also need to give the dummy consistently, every time you put him down during the first twenty-six weeks, because – confusingly – the evidence seems to indicate that babies are actually at greater risk of cot death if a dummy is routinely used, but then *not* given on a particular night. This places a great burden of responsibility on parents to *always* remember to make sure their baby has got his dummy for sleeping. Of course, if you don't want to give your baby a dummy at all, or if your baby isn't interested in one and simply spits it out when you offer it, this is one guideline you might reasonably, as parents, choose to remain relaxed about – particularly if you're scrupulously following all other advice on safe sleeping. If you feel unsure about this issue, then please do discuss it with your health visitor or GP.

What the netmums say

Dummy debates

I offered both of mine a dummy from day one. Joshua spat it out instantly and took no interest whatsoever in it, whilst Oliver, who was a very hungry, sucky baby, loved his. We used it to calm him in between feeds. Once weaning had started he began refusing his dummy, and hasn't had it since.
Maria from Bridgewater, mum to Joshua and Oliver, twenty-one months

We gave Jack a dummy when he was a couple of weeks old. I wasn't so keen but my husband thought it would help settle him and had heard it can reduce the risk of cot death, so I agreed in the end and I'm glad I did. I think a dummy is more hygienic than thumb-sucking and they're certainly easier to remove! Jack's dummy is long gone now, whilst my cousin in her twenties still sucks her thumb.
Vicky from Eastleigh, mum to Jack, three

With my eldest, I never offered a dummy. His dad was keen for me to use one, but I resisted, as he was a very content baby and I didn't think he needed one. My twins were in the neo-natal unit for over a week, and the staff there said a dummy would help with breastfeeding as it would help them develop their sucking reflex. Once we got them home, we started weaning them off the dummies and by the time they were ten weeks old they'd gone. In the meantime, I insisted on carrying around a small tub with steriliser solution in it to clean them.
Cat from Edinburgh, mum to George, six, and Freyja and Tavia, eleven months

We gave our daughter a dummy at about eight weeks after we decided to switch to formula feeding. She started off having it when she was upset or tired but as she got older she started to have it all the time. We've tried on several occasions to wean her off her dummy and for her to have it at nap times and bedtime, but this has proved unsuccessful. We're aiming for her to give it up before her third birthday.

Vikki from Northampton, mum to Bethany, two

I don't see the issues with dummies. Most children need some sort of comfort object, whether it's a dummy, a thumb or a cloth. They've even said now that they can possibly reduce the risk of cot death. Most children drop them of their own accord, and if they don't, then there are many strategies to wean them off. If it doesn't harm the child, and it's the difference between a full night's sleep or not, I know what I would choose.

Karen from Bradford, mum to William, six, and Joe, four

Having been determined to follow in my mum's footsteps and never use a dummy, I gave in at eight weeks. Thankfully it didn't affect breastfeeding as I'd feared it would. I took it away at fifteen months, before he could talk and ask me for it! I think every baby is different so I can't say I'd never use one again, but I think next time round I'd be more prepared for the crying fits and better equipped to handle them without a dummy.

Jenny from Oldham, mum to Oliver, twenty-one months

Personally I don't like dummies. I feel they're unhygienic, difficult to get rid of once they become a habit, and could interfere with speech. I deliberately avoided one in the early months because I was breastfeeding and didn't want to cause 'nipple confusion'. People would say my baby was using me as a substitute for a dummy, but I was always happy to provide that comfort.

Marianne from Uddingston, mum to William, twenty-two months

When I was pregnant I was determined never to offer a dummy and was set on breastfeeding for six months at least. But I had terrible problems getting breastfeeding established, which left my son frustrated and screaming all the time. The midwife suggested I calm him with a dummy and try again, and we found it was the one thing that could stop him crying.

Becky from Ashford, mum to Luca, two

As my son was in the neo-natal intensive care unit I was advised to give him a dummy to settle him. It haunts me four years on as he's obsessed with it still, although he has it a lot less now than he used to. I'm currently expecting and I don't plan to give this baby a dummy for at least the first six months while breastfeeding. And I hope I won't after that, to be honest.
Hayley from Staines, mum to Jay, four

I gave both my boys dummies and can't even bear to think what life would've been like without them! They both had really bad colicky digestive problems and cried for hours every day. Dummies helped them both sleep. We weaned Evan from his at five months. With Ashley, we only ever give it to him at sleep times so I'm not so worried about weaning him off it yet. Now that his gut is settling down I'll be weaning him off it soon. I don't understand why so many mums are so set against them. They're a lifesaver!
Alison from London, mum to Evan, two, and Ashley, five months

Breastfeeding was so painful, there was no way I was going to let him comfort suck on me, and the only way he would sleep was with my husband's little finger in his mouth, so we had no choice but to try a dummy. I was worried that he'd develop nipple confusion but he never had a problem switching between the two. He only has the dummy to sleep or if he's in his car seat or buggy, and crying. However, I have problems at night, having to get up to replace the dummy when he can't find it. I can't stand to see toddlers running round with a dummy in their mouths so at some point soon, I will only allow him to have it for sleeping.
Helena from York, mum to William, six months

I always said my child would not have a dummy, but never say 'never'! I gave Isabella one at about six weeks, as she needed the extra comfort. She still has it now, but she's also still breastfed, so it hasn't caused any problems there. She's only ever had it for naps and if she's really tired. I avoided giving it to her at bedtime as I didn't want to have her waking up at night when she lost it. People can be really snobbish about dummies. They carry a real stigma for some reason – I suppose there's the suggestion that you should be doing more to comfort your child. Personally I don't see the problem, unless it's permanently in their mouth.

Leanne from Bath, mum to Isabella, fourteen months

14 How do I know I'm feeding her enough?

Feeding your baby will no doubt be your number one priority in the early months – after all, it's in your natural instincts as a mum to ensure your little one is nourished and thriving. No wonder it's a major worry for parents who don't feel they're offering, or providing, the right amount of milk for their baby to grow at a healthy rate. For breastfeeding mums in particular, whilst there's rarely a fear of overfeeding to deal with, there's often anxiety that their baby is not getting enough milk. And formula feeding – whilst in some ways less of a worry, because at least you can calculate the amount going in – is not an exact science, either.

Whilst a few babies prompt genuine concern because they don't seem to be feeding or growing at the right rate, it's fair to say that most mums who worry about this issue do so needlessly. If, in the early months, you're being guided by your baby's demands, and the overall signs that she's thriving are in place, you've almost certainly got it right.

What the experts say

Louise says: A drawback of breastfeeding is that you can't see what's going in, which is why a lot of breastfeeding mums worry that their baby isn't getting enough milk. Another issue is that new babies will very often bring up what seems like a lot of milk after a feed (known as 'reflux'), which can lead you to wonder quite how much they managed to keep down. And many mums find it hard to believe quite how frequently a baby will feed in those early weeks: it's not unusual for a newborn to be on the boob as often as every hour. This is particularly so with a smaller baby, who will probably be able to take less and so may need to feed even more frequently. Mums can then misinterpret that, assuming their baby is not being satisfied. Sometimes they worry so much they offer formula as a top-up, and the result of that is that their supplies really do diminish, so they've got locked into a vicious circle.

The truth is that most mums really *can* produce enough milk to feed their babies sufficiently. Sometimes it just takes a while to feel confident about that. And it really is all about demand feeding during this period – if you allow your baby to feed whenever she seems to want to, breastfeeding's very clever supply-and-demand system means your milk should always replenish for the next time she needs it.

For some mums, there may be genuine concern about milk supply, and if a baby's health is at risk, then of course you'll prob-ably be advised to offer formula instead, or as a supplement. This may be disappointing if you were determined to breastfeed exclu-sively, and hopefully your feelings will have been taken into account, but as a rule it's best to be led by what the professionals say on this. Sucking or latch-on difficulties, or problems such as mastitis which make feeding impossibly painful, can also skew the supply and demand system. If you don't want to give up on breastfeeding, you may find it less painful to express and offer your milk in a bottle for a while.

The first few months are a time of rapid growth, and growth spurts may occur at various points, although it's by no means clear-cut as to when these occur. Your baby may want to feed more at these times and, if you want to be sure you're giving her enough, you may have to accept being pinned to the sofa for longer periods than usual. Give her whatever she needs if she genuinely seems hungrier than normal for a few days, but bear in mind a growth spurt is unlikely to last much longer than that.

If you're formula feeding, at least you know how much milk your baby's taking. But that doesn't mean it's obvious how much to offer – especially as it can vary so much according to weight, size and appetite, and the guideline charts on the back of tins can be very confusing. Just as with breastfeeding, it's best to be led by your baby. I'd say start off with a couple of ounces, and expect to offer it every two to four hours. What you want to be ending up with is a bottle that always has a little bit left in the bottom. You may have to accept there'll be some wastage at first. Once your baby's draining this much, and seems to be looking around for more after feeds, you can up it, an ounce at a time. It really is variable but in general, by three to four months, you'd expect to be offering around six 6 fl oz feeds a day. Whilst you can't really over-breastfeed, because breast milk comes ready-made to just the right composition for your baby's needs and isn't so calorie-dense, you *can* offer too much formula. It's a fact that some babies gain too much weight. To avoid this, be sure to make up feeds as advised on the tin. (And don't offer stage two or 'hungrier baby' varieties – even if you do think it could buy you a bit more sleep or a longer space in between feeds. They're not suitable for this age group, and can cause constipation.) Don't worry about wastage: if your baby's had enough of her formula feed, don't try to encourage her to take more. And watch that you're not using 'growth spurts' as an excuse for offering more formula than is necessary – it's fine to offer more for a few days if she really seems hungrier than usual, but bear in mind that these periods will usually only last a couple of days before settling back into a more normal pattern.

The best way to tell whether your baby's getting the right sort of quantity of milk – breast or formula – is to look at the overall picture. That means, firstly, is she producing lots of nappies for you to change? She should be making about six wet in every twenty-four-hour period. And regular poos are a good sign that all's well too – with a breastfed baby you may get several dirty nappies a day or fewer, and, typically, every one to two days if she is formula fed.

Your baby's weight gain will also be an important indicator that she's getting the right amount of food. It's impossible to say what's normal because every baby is different. But as a general rule – unless there were special medical circumstances – your midwife or health visitor will want your baby to have re-gained her birth weight in the first fortnight. And after that, she'll be looking for a rough but steady curve on the weight centile chart. It's no longer the norm for mums to take their babies to the clinic to be weighed every week, and this is no bad thing, as too much monitoring can actually increase anxiety! On the other hand, if there is cause for concern – or if you are worried that there may be – your health visitor should be happy to ensure your baby's weighed, and let you know if her progress is not as it should be. If you're a breast-feeding mum, bear in mind that your baby's weight gain probably won't be as speedy as her formula-fed contemporaries, and that, on average, breastfed babies tend to be a bit lighter.

The reassuring truth is that most worries about feeding will disappear after the first few months. Both breastfed and formula-fed babies will eventually settle into more regular schedules. More importantly still, your instincts kick in. You'll look at her and see that she's healthy, happy, and growing at what looks like the right rate. Then you'll know you're feeding her the right amount!

What the Netmums say

Milk monitoring

With my oldest, I was made to worry about how much milk he was getting by his dad, my ex. Harry struggled to breastfeed, so I decided to express milk for him, but my ex kept saying he wasn't getting enough – he even threw away the expressed breast milk I'd been sending when Harry visited him and gave him formula instead. I became increasingly paranoid that he wasn't getting enough and, after six months of expressing, I gave up. With my twins, I wasn't so worried. They were in neo-natal intensive care, and at the insistence of staff, they were given formula for the first thirty-six hours so they were getting the prescribed amount of milk when they needed it. But I managed to get breastfeeding established after that and I never had any worries. They were both gaining weight, and curious about the outside world. They still have two breastfeeds a day now.

Katie from Carlisle, mum to Harry, five, and Natalia and Isla, ten months

My first had problems with feeding and was in the neo-natal intensive care unit for three days being fed through a tube. It took him a long time to learn the sucking reflex, and we had to keep a chart on how much he was taking and how much he was keeping down. So, for the first couple of months it was very stressful until they signed him off and I was totally paranoid about whether he was getting enough. My second one suffered with reflux, so after gulping down 6 fl oz of milk he would then throw up two-thirds of it. However, he still gained weight and produced plenty of dirty nappies, so I wasn't too worried.

Fae from Basildon, mum to Alexander, four, and Nicholas, seventeen months

I breastfed both my babies beyond a year and I never worried how much they were getting. I never even got them weighed after the first couple of checks. I just figured that my body would provide my babies with what they needed. I've always fed on demand, however often that may be, and they've thrived. I could never express more than about five ounces, though. Hence I never used bottles and so have never been able to go out!

Camilla from Ipswich, mum to Savannah, two, and Willow, six months

Megan was bottle-fed from day one, but she was a big baby and, as stupid as it sounds now, we were never sure whether to follow the amount of formula the jar said for her weight or for her age. At first we were going by what it said for her age rather than her weight, and obviously she wasn't getting enough. So over several days we upped the quantity gradually, in case we gave her too much and she just threw it back up again. We worried about everything, instead of just following our instincts! We did eventually get the hang of it but we didn't get her weighed that regularly and so had to wait for her to tell us that she wasn't getting enough – which was what we assumed was happening once she was draining her bottles and then seemed to want feeding again in less time than we'd expected – so then we knew we needed to up the amount of feed. Having said that, though, she would often feed quite slowly so it wasn't always clear if she was hungry or if she was just taking the milk because it was there. And sometimes we'd just get into a good feeding routine and she'd have a growth spurt and the whole routine would go out of the window and we'd have to start afresh again. She's a happy, healthy three-year-old now, so it all worked out right in the end!

Catherine from Preston, mum to Megan, three

I breastfed my eldest daughter and she seemed to want to feed constantly, so I worried that maybe I wasn't producing enough milk. My health visitors just said the more you feed, the more you'll produce. I tried really hard to keep going but by week nine I'd had enough. I didn't feel it was worth it because I couldn't be the mummy I wanted to be, as all I was doing was sleeping or feeding. So I gradually weaned her off me and on to the bottle. It was the best decision I made as my energy came back and I could begin enjoying my baby. I weaned my second baby on to the bottle at ten weeks, too.

Stephanie from Rochdale, mum to Emily, four, and Lilly, two

At first my son seemed to be feeding well. But by four days old he'd lost eleven per cent of his body weight. That night Max screamed all night, wouldn't go down, and wanted feeding constantly. The next morning the midwife weighed him again and discovered he'd lost more weight still, and was jaundiced. We went into hospital for three days and were encouraged by the midwives there to introduce formula as a top-up. So I would breastfeed Max, then give him a syringe of expressed milk, and then hand him over to my hubbie to bottle-feed him while I expressed more. His weight improved dramatically and the jaundice disappeared. Five weeks, on I'm still breastfeeding and topping up with formula but I've dropped the expressing as it was stressing me out and not particularly productive. Max has no problem switching between breast and bottle, although the HVs say that at some point he'll just prefer the bottle and won't want my boob any more. I'll be sad when that happens. But I'm too scared to try just breastfeeding on its own again as I still don't think I have enough milk – I've never felt engorged, and I don't really need breast pads as I don't ever leak.

There's no information out there about what happens or what to do if you don't have a lot of milk.
Helen from Bristol, mum to Max, six weeks

My first son spent the beginning of his life in the SCBU and when he came home I bottle-fed him expressed milk so I knew exactly how much he was getting, and I never worried that he wasn't having enough milk. He often stopped before emptying the bottle, anyway. I breastfed my second son and at first I struggled to understand how much he was getting. He would always feed for less than ten minutes, and his poo was slightly green, which an internet search suggested was down to him getting too much foremilk and not enough hind milk. I've reasoned he must be getting enough of both, though, because he's already growing faster than I expected. He's now settled into an on-demand routine and is sleeping in two five-hour blocks through the night with a ten-minute feed in between. Presumably he's getting enough, otherwise he'd be waking up complaining about the poor service!
Lucy from Croydon, mum to Morgan, three, and Lincoln, three months

I started to breastfeed my daughter from day one but after a week my health visitor told me she wasn't putting on enough weight. After a fortnight she still wasn't back to her birth weight, and I was advised to give her formula. I agreed to express and top up with formula if needed, even though my health visitor predicted, rather harshly, that I would give up expressing after a week and go on to formula. I did manage to carry on expressing until she was four months so that at least two-thirds of her daily intake was breast milk. Even then I felt like a failure as I wondered if I could have done more to breastfeed exclusively.
Monica from Farnham, mum to Eva, fifteen months

Breastfeeding was a real struggle initially. My little one didn't want to make the effort of latching on until my milk came through properly on day five, by which time he was yellow and quite listless. I had to express milk and feed it to him, but as soon as the 'real stuff' came through, he quickly learnt how to get what he wanted for himself! I didn't worry too much initially as he was a healthy birth

weight and once my milk did come through, I had gallons of the stuff. He's still exclusively breastfed and as he's getting chunky, I'm happy he's getting enough milk. I'm not worried about him having too much, either. I'm sure as soon as he starts moving around more by himself, the weight will come back off. I've heard of some mums saying they're worried about their baby getting enough milk and then their milk has dried up, and I wonder if there's a link between getting stressed and tired, and the quality of their milk going down. If you were worried, and tempted to offer formula instead, you would presumably start producing less milk as a result.
Sophie from Aberdeen, mum to Joshua, four months

I wanted to breastfeed but after five days it seemed obvious to me that something wasn't right. I was in hospital after an emergency C-section and the midwives assured me the latch-on was right, but I felt sure she was hungry and was just not getting enough milk from me. I gave her a bottle and she guzzled it down and slept soundly for the first time since being born, so I continued to bottle-feed, to the obvious disappointment of the staff. However, once back home, the community midwife said she was appalled that my baby had lost so much weight. I'm extremely glad I followed my instincts and gave her that bottle. Within another week she'd gone back to her birth weight and is now a happy, smiley, content little girl.
Louisa from Cannock, mum to Darcey, five months

I always believed that my body would produce exactly what my babies needed, and it did. I breastfed them exclusively, on demand, for seven months, then continued mixed feeding until they were a year old, since both first and second time round, pregnancy decreased my supply. The only time I had doubts was when a health visitor told me I had to start giving my second son baby rice at seventeen weeks because he hadn't put on as much weight as he 'should have'. I'd planned to begin baby-led weaning at six months and wasn't happy with this advice so I continued exclusive breastfeeding, and his weight was fine at the next weigh-in! I'm glad I trusted my instincts. I had no idea about growth spurts as a first-time mum, but after going through a nightmare few weeks with my first son when he was about four months old, I found out

that it's a common time for this. With the benefit of experience, I knew when my second and third sons were going through a demanding patch that I just had to keep on offering the breast whenever they seemed to need it, until things settled down again.
Ingrid from Warwick, mum to Jadon, three, Caleb, twenty-one months, and Bram, four months

My son just would not suck, and I ended up bottle-feeding with formula from day two. I did give expressing a try when my milk came, but it just took too long. However I feel there's little or no support and nowhere to turn to for questions when you're formula feeding. I had no idea what formula to use, and no idea how much he should be having (he was 9 lb 5 oz at birth which was almost the equivalent of two to four months of age, according to the formula tin guidelines). When I asked the midwife, I was told the minimum they'd expect a baby to be on, and that was it. At about seven weeks, I asked my HV again how much milk she'd expect him to be on, as he was demand-feeding every two hours. She just said he was a hungry baby and not to worry, but when the doctor saw his notes I was accused of overfeeding him and advised to stretch the time in between feeds from two hours to three. As my son wasn't always draining his bottles I assumed he was self-regulating, so I continued to offer him a feed when he seemed to want it. I feel the formula-tin guidelines seem way too low. For his age and weight, they recommend 6 fl oz bottles five times a day, but even though he's more or less sleeping through the night, he'll still have seven bottles or more a day. And as he's in between the seventy-fifth and ninety-first centile, he's not overweight.
Emma from Banbury, mum to Nathaniel, four months

15 Why is he crying so much?

Crying is completely normal in babies – it's how they communicate their needs to their parents. Usually, you'll be able to calm your baby's cries by addressing the various possibilities until you can meet with a solution: is he hungry, tired, in need of a fresh nappy, or simply fed up, and looking for a cuddle? You'll probably start to recognise different cries, and eventually develop a schedule which means you'll usually know what he needs, and when. Until then, you may just have to run through the options for comfort, until you hit on the right one.

As many as one in five babies cry excessively, inconsolably, and without any obvious reason. Sometimes, there'll turn out to be a medical reason for a baby who's crying a lot. But mostly, there won't. If your baby has long bouts of crying which you can't seem to calm, typically at its worst in the late afternoon or evening, he probably has infant colic – not a condition as such, but a broad term that defines bouts of excessive crying in an otherwise healthy baby. Any parent who's had to cope with colic – particularly for the first time – will tell you it was a nightmare. With no explanation for it, no certain cure, and no idea of how long it will go on for, it can be a miserable time all round. The reassuring truth is that colic is almost always a phase that's consigned to history within three or four months, although unfortunately, at the time, it can seem like a great deal longer.

What the experts say

Maggie says: No one knows for sure what causes colic, although there are several theories. One is that it's a result of abdominal pain, caused by excess wind or an immature digestive system. Another is that babies may suffer from a 'permanent headache' caused by structural stress on the brain, as a consequence of birth. Other schools of thought suggest a colicky baby is simply 'out of sorts' with the world and still adapting to life outside the womb, or suffering from a sensory overload at the end of a long day. Some say that babies who cry a lot are picking up anxiety from their parents. What we do know is that it's very common and that in most cases it's a phase with no obvious cause, which will be over within three months – perhaps a little longer, if you're unlucky. Until then, it's basically a question of finding ways to get through it. However, I would advise getting your baby checked out by a doctor before assuming his crying is caused by harmless colic. I know some doctors can be rather unsympathetic because colic's such a common thing. But he or she should be able to rule out any more significant potential causes.

Although there are no cures for colic, there are many different things to try that might help. What works for one baby may not for another, and you'll more than likely have to use a process of trial and error to find out what works for yours. All three of my children suffered from it as babies, and I found that putting them on their backs and massaging their tummies or moving their legs in a bicycling motion seemed to stop the crying, if only for a while.

Lots of colicky babies respond to motion of some sort. You could try walking up and down the stairs, or gently rocking or jiggling him. A solution that works for lots of parents is to put him in the pram or sling and go for a walk or take him for a drive in the car. Certain noises are said to help, usually those that emulate the conditions of the womb, so the rhythmic churning of a washing machine, a ticking clock, or specifically recorded 'womb music' can help. And music generally can have a soothing effect – one survey actually found Brahms and Bach to be particularly effective!

Lots of colicky babies are comforted by sucking, so you could try offering a breast or a dummy. If you're bottle-feeding, it might help to keep the bottle upright and make sure the neck of the bottle is always covered in milk, to reduce the chance of wind. And if you're breastfeeding, bear in mind the theory that your baby may be sensitive to something in your diet – wheat, dairy, caffeine, citrus fruits, alcohol and strong veg such as cauliflower are said to be likely culprits. You could try keeping a food diary and cutting things out in turn to see if there's any improvement.

Herbal remedies might be worth a try and as they're natural and harmless, you've nothing to lose. Camomile, fennel and peppermint teas, available from reputable health-food shops or big chemists, are recommended for colic. Offer one teaspoon to your baby on a teaspoon or diluted in a bottle of water, or drink a cup yourself if breastfeeding. Another 'alternative' treatment for crying babies is cranial osteopathy, which it's said can help re-shape and reduce pressure on the skull. There's no real evidence that it works and you'll have to go private if you want to try it, as it's not available on the NHS. However, anecdotally, many parents report results.

If nothing else, trying out different solutions can make you feel like at least you're doing something, which can help take your mind off the crying until the phase passes – which it will, eventually.

Dr David says: Colic is something that affects a lot of babies and in most cases, it will be something you and your baby have to live with until the phase passes. However, if it's persistent crying which lasts for more than three hours a day, on more than three days a week, which lasts for at least three weeks, then it's important to check with your GP in case there's a medical problem which can be treated.

One possible cause is cow's milk allergy, although if this is the case, you're likely to notice other symptoms beyond just crying, for example slow weight gain, bloody poo, or eczema. If your doctor suspects an allergy and you're breastfeeding he'll probably advise you to cut cows' milk out of your diet for four to six weeks to see if it helps, and if your baby's bottle-fed, he's likely to suggest trying a hypoallergenic formula, available only on prescription, for the same period of time. Reintroducing dairy products or normal formula will then confirm whether either is causing the problem or not. *Never* be tempted to diagnose an allergy yourself, though, or attempt to offer an alternative like soya milk, which isn't suitable for young babies under six months, and can cause an allergic reaction in itself. Lactose-free milk will not help with cow's milk allergy, either, as it contains the same protein.

Gastro-oesophageal reflux is a symptom that is very normal in young babies and is often blamed for discomfort and excessive crying. It occurs because the oesophageal sphincter is under-developed in the early months, which means the top of the stomach remains loose, allowing its contents to reflux back up into the oesophagus, or food pipe. It's worth seeing your GP if you suspect reflux may be a problem, although the reality is that there's little evidence that medication will definitely help, and the vast majority of children grow out of it by one to two years of age, once they're eating more solids and spending more time upright. Sometimes, doctors will prescribe a feed thickener such as Infant Gaviscon, which can help milk to stay put in the stomach, or suggest switching to a special formula that works in the same way.

A sudden onset of crying that's different to your baby's normal crying behaviour is something that should ring alarm bells as it could be caused by an infection or other serious problem – particularly if it's accompanied by fever, reluctance to feed, vomiting or sleepiness. Get it checked out straight away.

Crissy says: I've heard it said that the average healthy baby cries for anything up to three hours every day. Incredibly, a baby's cry can actually cause his parents' resting heart rates to double, so there's no doubt it can provoke considerable anxiety and agitation. With no apparent explanation or solution at your fingertips, and an inconsolable baby in your arms, you'll be facing one of the most stressful challenges of early parenthood. The sheer torment of a relentlessly crying baby can leave you feeling fearful, frustrated, and even furious – not exactly the tender loving emotions you anticipated feeling towards your new baby, but entirely understandable nonetheless. Ironically, to make matters worse, chances are your baby will pick up on your anxiety and be even harder to pacify as a result.

Persistent crying can shred both your nerves and your confidence. When all his physical needs have been met, you've ruled out any potential health issues and no amount of cuddling has made a difference it's tempting to blame yourself for your baby's distress, and so it's hardly surprising in the heat of the moment if you feel like screaming or running away. Pushed to their utmost limits even the most devoted parents may feel like shouting, rough handling or even shaking their baby, but if you ever find yourself on the edge of causing your baby harm in any way, put him in a safe place like his cot or pram, and leave the room. He won't come to any harm during the few moments you're away but it will give you time to take a deep breath, regain your composure and if necessary, seek help. You may find that some time out for a quick cuppa, a chat with your neighbour or a brisk walk in the park with your baby in the sling or buggy is all you need to calm things down. But if you're feeling overwhelmed and struggling to cope you may need a longer break, some proper time alone, or maybe a nap. This is where mum's best friend is her phone. Ask someone you trust to come over and take care of your baby for a while, or if there's no one available or you feel uncomfortable asking someone you know, consider calling a specialist helpline like CRY-SIS or Family Lives (formerly Parentline Plus) for emotional support and advice. Sometimes connecting with another adult and hearing an understanding voice at the other end of the line can make all the difference. Wherever possible ask for help when you need it rather than when you've already reached breaking point. All mums need some time apart from their babies so don't wait to be asked, be proactive and enlist the help of family and friends to support you in taking some regular 'me time'.

If you're suffering from postnatal depression or have other mental health issues and the crying is compounding them, or if you fear that you or your baby are at risk of harm, it's essential that you find a way to ask for help as soon as possible. This is not the time to suffer in silence. If speaking to a health professional feels too daunting at first, start by opening up to someone close to you such as your partner, a family member or good friend.

What the netmums say

Coping with cry-babies

For the first three months, sunset was hellish. Erin cried for about half an hour every day, and always at that time of day. The midwife said it was colic, my mother-in-law said she obviously didn't like the night drawing in! Either way, I felt helpless. The only way to soothe her was for me to sit on my yoga ball with her body upright, held against my chest, and gently bounce up and down. Erin would fall asleep – and I developed thighs like steel!
Nicki from Sandgate, mum to Erin, five, Jack, two, and Sam, twenty-two months

My son hardly ever cried, but my daughter cried over the tiniest thing constantly until she was about eight or nine months. She never seemed to be in pain, and it was a strange shouty cry, but we sought help and tried everything as we were so worried about her. Looking back now, we wonder if it was at least partly because of her personality. She's the polar opposite of her quiet, laid-back brother. I can see her becoming a stubborn, driven, passionate girl who knows her own mind. Perhaps that contributed to all the crying, who knows?
Carolann from Dundee, mum to Dominic, three, and Matilda, fourteen months

The only thing that settles my son is breastfeeding. For the first five months of his life he was rarely out of my arms or my husband's, or the sling. Gripe water helped a bit. We took him to the chiropractor when he was a few weeks old and they found some tightness on his back but even after the treatment the colic continued. We've also started some cranial osteopathy. It's now much easier to tell what he wants when he's crying. And a breastfeed always sorts him out. The crying hasn't bothered me particularly, but it's hard not knowing what the problem is. I've come to the conclusion he just likes cuddles!
Jane from Poole, mum to Eleanor, two, and Stanley, seven months

My wee man used to cry all the time unless he was being nursed or held. It turned out the cause was an undiagnosed milk allergy that corrected itself once I cut dairy out of my diet. I found nursing him when he was upset for comfort and holding him or carrying him around made him feel better. Unfortunately I got a lot of stick from other people because they would say I was spoiling him, or that he was just using me as a dummy, or even that he was nursing all the time because my milk wasn't enough for him and that I should give formula (which actually would have had horrible conse- quences, because of the allergy).
Marianne from Uddingston, mum to William, twenty-two months

Nathan cried every day, for most of the day. He wanted to be held and cuddled all the time – it was hard work. I tried cranial osteopathy and it didn't work, so we just put it down to colic. Once he could crawl and walk he improved a lot. My youngest was the same, she would scream for hours on end. Nothing would console her, we just used to walk around with her or push her in the pram until she fell asleep. I tried everything available to treat colic and nothing worked, and went to the doctor's repeatedly as my instincts were telling me it was not colic, but I got nowhere. Treatment for reflux didn't make much difference. Finally I insisted they refer her to a paediatrician who put her on a hypoallergenic formula, and almost instantly the screaming stopped. Now I can't help but wonder whether my youngest son had the same problem. I still feel angry that my concerns were dismissed for so long.
Sarah from Wirral, mum to Kieran, fourteen, Matthew, five, Nathan, four, and Freya, seven months

My little boy cried continuously for the first three months. My health visitor recommended a cranial osteopath and after three sessions he was like a different baby. The cranial osteopath thought it was because he was born back-to-back and therefore there would have been a lot of pressure on his head, likening it to him having a permanent headache.
Clair from Penrith, mum to Osker, three

James was what others politely called a 'grisly' baby. He cried or moaned unless he was asleep, on the breast or being walked around the room. The only thing that would always settle him was putting him on the breast – I became a human dummy! It wasn't until he would sit up at around seven months that he became content to amuse himself. He's now a fantastic, happy little boy who plays really well on his own. My second son, Alex, was the opposite; he only really cried if he needed something, and yet he's the one now who wants us to play with him and craves attention. I don't really understand it.

Jenny from Coventry, mum to James, four, and Alex, two

Ewan has cried excessively since day one, and still cries a lot. I find the crying exhausting, particularly since his sleeping is also very erratic and I'm now back at work. Holding him and walking around the room seems to be the only way to settle him, but I also have a four-year-old daughter so this can be very difficult. It's put strain on the whole family, and sometimes feels like it's never going to end.

Linda from East Kilbride, mum to Amy, four, and Ewan, nine months

The first three months were agony as my daughter cried and cried. One day I timed it, and she cried for eight out of twelve hours. The only time she didn't cry was when she was upright on one of our chests. I went to the GP many times only to be told it was colic. After three long months, she was diagnosed with acid reflux. Once we got some medication and were told not to put her down flat on her back, things improved. Looking back it was obvious it was reflux and I feel bitter that we all had to go through those first precious months with her in constant pain. Unfortunately, not all health professionals pick up on the signs soon enough.

Sarah from Nottingham, mum to Mia, seven

16 Should we be in a routine?

Routine is a word you may hear a lot when your baby is young – in particular, a lot of people may promise you that once you've got one of these in place, your life will be a lot easier. Chances are, in those blurred early weeks, you'll find yourself wondering when and if your baby will take to waking, feeding, napping, playing and going down for the evening at the same sort of times every day – and what you can do to hasten it!

When it comes to routine, it's a case of different strokes for different folks. Most parents agree that some sort of flexible routine makes for an easier life, and will usually make for a happier baby. Some think a rigid routine, usually implemented early on, is better still. Others prefer to chill out totally when it comes to timings, and take a 'baby-led' approach. Whichever school of thought you subscribe to, it's worth knowing that pretty much all babies slot into a natural routine of sorts over time. Whether or not you choose to exploit that is down to you.

What the experts say

Louise says: There's no doubt that some sort of routine can make for an easier time – if you know roughly when your baby is going to need feeding, or likely to get tired and want a nap, you can plan your day more effectively. And most babies, quite naturally, prefer the security of getting what they want, when they want it – as you've no doubt discovered on days when a feed or a sleep was later than it ought to have been.

However, I always say there's not a lot of point in worrying about routine in the first month or two. Most new mums find their baby's sleeping, waking and feeding times are just 'all over the place' at first and that a baby-led approach is the only option. You may also feel quite dazed enough catering to her needs without having to do so to schedule.

One early step you *can* take in helping a routine develop is aiming to differentiate between day and night, and you can do this as early as you feel able. So, get your baby up and dressed in the morning, make sure the curtains are open and keep things lively and sociable when she's awake, and put her down for naps in a room that's not particularly dark and where there'll be some background noise. Then at bedtime, and when she wakes in the night, try to keep things very quiet, calm and boring, and the lights dim.

With or without your encouragement, your baby will almost certainly start to adopt a routine eventually. Usually you'll notice patterns starting to emerge, quite naturally, once the dust settles and you've got those chaotic early months under your belt, and when that happens you can capitalise on it by following the pattern, aiming to plan your day so you can offer feeds or put her down for a nap at the same sort of time from then on. It's important to keep feeding on demand in the first three months or so, but once past this point you can certainly aim for a more regular feeding schedule if she hasn't already slotted into one. Three to four-hourly will be typical, by then, but you may have to space out feeds if she's used to getting one more often than that. Be prepared to distract her in between if she's not too chuffed about it, with play, a cuddle, or a walk.

One element of routine that *is* worth being proactive about getting in place as soon as you can is a regular bedtime, with a consistent preamble that involves some quiet, calming time and – typically – a bath, feed and cuddle before putting her down. As well as being a primary step in establishing an overall schedule, all the experts agree that it's a really healthy habit, because it sets up lots of good sleep associations or 'cues' for your baby, which will help pave the way to a whole night's sleep a bit later down the line. In fact, it's a habit you're likely to be very grateful you started, as it will help you avoid bedtime battles for years to come. It also means that you can have the evening to yourselves, which, while not a necessity for all parents, is considered a real boon by many.

Plenty of people swear by getting a rigid routine in place from day one, as prescribed by certain baby-care experts. The drawback of these is that you have to be disciplined and committed to make them work, and you can rather become a slave to them. I also suspect they may hinder mums from getting in tune with their babies during those precious early weeks. You may feel that's a pay-off worth making. At the other end of the spectrum, a completely carefree, baby-led approach, in which routines are not required at all, may be your preference. If that way of life suits you, your family and your baby, go for it!

What the netmums say

Schedule versus go-with-the-flow

I followed the midwife and health visitor's advice on feeding times, but other than that we let our little one fall into her own 'routine'. At five months old she now has a set routine that she dictates and which suits all of us. She eats at roughly the same time every day and has her naps and play times around the same time too so we all know where we are! I think very strict routines that are supposed to be implemented from birth are totally impractical.
Liz from Penzance, mum to Ellora, five months

My feeling is that babies aren't meant to have a routine, particularly when it comes to feeding. We eat when we're hungry, why should we make our babies wait until we say it's time to feed? We've sort of naturally fallen into some sort of routine – bath between 6.30–7.30, story, and bed at about 9 p.m., sleep by 10 p.m. We've never really intentionally done that, it just seems to have happened. With no set bedtime, you never have to have a

fight. I think we all need to chill out a bit with our babies and go with it. As parents we're always trying to mould our children around our lives, instead of moulding our lives around our children. Then when something doesn't go right, it's stressful!
Marianne from Uddingston, mum to William, twenty-two months

A bit of both has worked for my two, and they've both fed and slept well. You can't set yourself too much of a routine in the first few months, otherwise you end up putting too much pressure on yourself. When kids are hungry they let you know and when they are tired they let you know! I established a good sleeping routine with mine from about eight weeks, allowing them one nap in the morning and one in the afternoon. Every child is different and every mummy is different so you go with what works for you, but my advice is don't put any pressure on yourself and trust your instincts.
Evie from Manchester, mum to Isobel, six, and Jacob, sixteen months

We just went with it. I breastfeed, so did that on demand. We didn't start giving him baths for a month, and then it was every couple of days. At about two months we started a bedtime routine that we still use now. Eventually he got himself in some kind of schedule – feeding every two hours, waking up, and napping at similar times every day. I found the *Baby Whisperer* book, and loosely followed the advice about routines in that. I'm quite happy the way we have done it, but he is an easy baby so I think that helps.
Clare from London, mum to Josh, six months

For the most part, I just went with the flow – let her nap when she was tired, fed her when she was hungry, and played with her the rest of the time – except at bedtimes, when she's always had a routine, from the night I brought her home. Bath, bottle, story, snuggles, bed. Even now, although she's dropped the bottle, we still do it just the same. She's always gone down without any tears, whoever puts her to bed. In fact, on the odd occasion where we've lost track of time, she will let us know it's time for her bath herself!
Karin from Watford, mum to Kayleigh, two

Routine all the way for me. I have been more relaxed with my third daughter, but she has slotted into the routine that was already in place for the older two. I realised very early on, having twins, that if I didn't establish a routine then I would not have a life outside of feeding and changing nappies. I used Gina Ford as a rough guide only, and never left them to cry if they were hungry or woke them up if they were sleeping, but I consciously stuck to feed and sleep times whenever I could. They are all very happy, contented girls who eat and sleep well, and so it has worked for us.
Mel from Manchester, mum to Paige and Grace, four, and Willow, eighteen months

We are living proof that routines are not necessary or even particularly beneficial! I fed my eldest whenever she wanted it as a baby and I now do the same for my youngest, although thankfully she feeds a lot less frequently. I've had both in bed with me and, as I could never see the point in putting a young baby to bed at 7 p.m., only to be woken at 6 a.m., I've always just taken them when I go at 11 p.m. I accept that a routine becomes necessary a bit later, and I've already brought Savannah's bedtime forward which I did with no problems, over the course of a week, to 8.30 p.m. I'll bring it forward again once playgroup approaches. She's now in a routine that developed naturally. Hopefully Willow will make the same changes easily when the time comes. Although a lot of people question my parenting, I now have two very content, independent children. Happy kids, happy mum.
Camilla from Ipswich, mum to Savannah, two, and Willow, six months

My son had no routine at first and it was awful. We then went with my nan's advice on strict feeding and putting down times. Within a week he was sleeping through and had gone from being a windy, crying baby to a happy one. Lesson learnt. When I was pregnant again I came across Gina Ford. She seemed to have the same ideas as my nan, who sadly had since died, so I bought the book. We did it from day one and found when we followed it life was fab, but when we stopped she got over-tired and whingy. From sixteen weeks, she was sleeping twelve hours a night and

four in the day, and she still sleeps brilliantly now.
Shelley from Hastings, mum to Callum, three, and Leila, eleven months

Isaac had a cleft palate so I expressed his feeds – and trust me, you have to have an element of routine to manage that! However, I tried to go on demand as far as possible, and allowed sleep to be led by him. I honestly believe that children will naturally find a routine that suits them. With my daughter, I breastfed for six months, and found that she dropped into a routine very quickly. The only thing I deliberately changed was her was bedtime. She was dropping into a natural 9 p.m. bedtime and I wanted her down at 7 p.m! I would recommend allowing a child to find their own rhythm. However, all parents need some elements in life that are predictable – like bedtime, sleep and mealtimes, so I don't think that simply allowing the child to determine everything is right either. Neither extreme is best.
Anna from Newton Abbot, mum to Isaac, three, and Milly, two

With my eldest, Alice, we didn't try to establish a routine at all, and she never really got herself into one. For most of her first two years it was just me and her, so it wasn't a problem as far as I was concerned. By the time Byron came along we had established a routine for Alice and it made sense to fit him into the same schedule. The same has happened with my third, who goes to bed when his brother and sister do. I now really value having the evening as child-free time, and I've found that bedtimes go more smoothly with a regular pattern.
Abi from Mitcham, mum to Alice, eight, Byron, five, and Phoenix, eight months

I found a strict routine was a huge help. Before having my little girl I was pro the 'baby-led' approach. However, I found on-demand feeding and sleeping did not work out. Victoria lost weight, never settled, cried continuously and did not feed well. In desperation, after three weeks of 'going with the flow', I started using the Gina Ford book, which a friend had given me. Within a day I had a much happier baby who slept and fed well, which allowed me to relax and enjoy her. And far from being restrictive, I found it made getting out and about easier as I knew what she would be doing or what she would need at any time of the day. At nine weeks she slept through the night. For me, having a routine and clear instructions to follow, at a time when tiredness makes decision-making very difficult, was a lifesaver.

Alison from Bristol, mum to Victoria, twenty-one months

All babies are different and what works for one won't necessarily for another. I have friends who stick to a prescribed routine rigidly and as a result absolutely will not or can't do things that may interfere with it! But what's the worst that can happen if your baby has lunch at 1 p.m. instead of 12.30? Babies have a way of finding their own pattern of doing things and people who think they don't have a 'routine' probably do, it's just not a strict schedule! We started off going with flow and demand feeding for first few months and eventually my daughter fell into her own routine, with a little help. Now we have a kind of routine but it certainly doesn't prevent us doing things and as a result she's a very flexible little girl.

Leanne from Bath, mum to Isabella, fourteen months

17 Was that a smile, or wind?

It's the milestone achievement that's most likely to warm a parent's heart. But when will your baby break into his first smile: and how do you know he hasn't just got gas?

As well as being a happy moment, your baby's early smiles are developmentally significant because they show that he is responding to *your* smiles, and to other stimuli, such as your voice. He'll learn how to smile by copying you, so the best thing you can do to encourage it is to beam at him whenever you get the chance. Don't worry if your baby is a late starter on the smiling front. Anything up to three months is normal, and if he was born pre-term, remember – as with all the milestones – to adjust your expectations accordingly.

What the experts say

Louise says: Technically, babies can 'smile' from the start – in fact, thanks to ultrasound technology we know they smile sometimes in utero – but for the first couple of weeks, it won't be true smiling but a reflex action, usually when he's asleep or wind-stricken, hence the traditional explanation for those early grins. However, once your baby has smiled 'by accident' and he picks up on the positive response it gets him, it won't be long before he's smiling with meaning – on average, at between four and eight weeks old. Some parents are quite convinced they've seen a proper smile even before that – and perhaps they have! You'll know when it's a real smile rather than a reflex action, because his whole face will light up.

Your GP may ask if your baby is smiling yet at his six-week check-up, but anything up to about twelve weeks is a normal timeframe for this milestone. In the unlikely event that your baby isn't smiling after that, you'd be wise to mention it to a health professional.

Crissy says: Many mums recall fondly the moment when their baby graced them with his first real smile. Amid the hustle and bustle of those early weeks, reaching this often long-awaited milestone may feel like a welcome reward for all those sleepless nights and can reassure new mums that they really are getting it right and that their baby does love them after all. Although this first smile may be somewhat of a happy accident, the pleasure your baby experiences in your joyful response teaches him that smiles breed smiles and can therefore bring him the warmth and attention he needs. At first these social smiles may be rather indiscriminately bestowed, but in time he will learn to save his biggest and brightest for you.

Because babies are capable of attuning to their mother's mood and state of mind, it is possible that an infant's emotional development may be hindered or impaired in some way when a mum (perhaps because she's experiencing emotional, physical or social difficulties) persistently over time feels unable to fully engage with her baby. But if you're struggling to return your baby's smiles and that special mother/baby bond is taking far longer than you expected to develop, don't despair. Babies do need attentive, consistent and attuned care but it doesn't need to come exclusively from you. In the short term, as long as someone close to your baby is delivering those smiles – whether it's his dad, siblings, relatives or friends, your baby will be OK. So turn that parenting pressure valve down and turn your attention instead to finding ways to access the help and support you need right now to feel better.

What the netmums say

Give us a smile

Jack's first smile was unmistakeable. He was five weeks old and sitting on my lap, being gently bounced on my knee. He looked straight into my eyes and opened his mouth wide. His eyes lit up and I could see the pure joy in his face. I felt so proud. Unfortunately his dad was at work, and extremely disappointed to have missed it.
Lisa from London, mum to Jack, four months

Joseph first smiled at four weeks. Although everyone said it was wind, I knew it wasn't. It wasn't until he smiled at my other half that people believed us, as they realised we couldn't both be wrong! It's amazing.
Laura from Aldershot, mum to Joseph, four months

I think Megan was six or seven weeks old, although it's hard to remember exactly now. I do remember that we were unsure whether she was smiling or if it was wind the first time she did it but the next day she gave us lots of very definite smiles and since it happened to be Mother's Day, I prefer to think that her first real smile was then!
Catherine from Preston, mum to Megan, three

William's first smile came at six weeks. We were at Mum and Dad's house and we'd been trying for about a week to get a grin out of him. In the end it was the dog coming up to him and licking his face that did it – he let out a big chuckle, which had us giggling too. Samantha smiled for the first time at five weeks, thanks to a tickle from her granddad.
Vikki from Bradford, mum to William, three, and Samantha, seven months

We were told that smiles before about six weeks were always wind, but we are sure that's not always true as from two to three weeks we definitely had the first tentative smiles from our son. We could

tell the difference between 'gas smiling' and proper smiling because his trumps are noisy and they smell! He now smiles all the time, particularly when he recognises certain people – his daddy, grandma and auntie. It's just lovely to see their reactions.
Clare from Portsmouth, mum to Edward, three months

My daughter's first smiles were at two to three weeks, when she used to smile in her sleep. Yes, I know people say it's wind. But she was doing this full-on, big cheesy smile! It melted my heart. At six weeks she smiled for the first time awake. She was just sitting on my lap and I was talking to her when this huge big grin lit up her whole face! It was the most amazing feeling in the world.
Robyn from Harrogate, mum to Teagan, three months

Zahra first smiled at us at two weeks old. Some people said it wasn't possible, but we knew she had smiled. She did it for her grandma, too, at three weeks. We managed to catch it on camera so we had proof. Her smiles are always in response to people she knows when she first sees and hears them – a kind of 'I know and like you' smile! She now has a little laugh every so often, too.
Susannah from Manchester, mum to Zahra, three months

I can't exactly remember when my babies smiled for the first time, but it was earlier than they say it should be – maybe three or four weeks. And as my other half sagely pointed out, if they can look bloomin' miserable from birth, why shouldn't they be smiling that early on, too?!
Hannah from Newcastle, mum to Ted, seven, Kip, five, and Annis, two

Nathaniel was five weeks old. I'd spent a few days asking some of my online mummy friends how they knew it was a proper smile, and they said I'd just know, as it was a smile that reached their eyes. I realised then I'd actually missed one. Luckily he did it pretty soon again afterwards and yes, it was a 'whole-face' smile. Now he smiles all the time, at everyone – especially cameras!
Emma from Banbury, mum to Nathaniel, four months

18 How do I cut her nails?

It's a task that makes many new parents wince – trimming those tiny but surprisingly long little fingernails, without nicking the soft skin behind or causing even worse damage when she pulls her little hand away. But's it's a job that's hard to avoid, because your little one may be scratching her face badly – and maybe you too, particularly if she likes to grab a handful of boob while breastfeeding. You've probably found there aren't many helpful alternatives – those cute little scratch mitts you probably bought in preparation for her arrival rarely stay put. So it really is a case of needs must.

Try to relax about cutting her nails. You need the right equipment and a steady hand. If in doubt, wait until your baby's out for the count before trying. And if you really can't bear it, ask someone else to do the deed!

What the experts say

Louise says: You probably won't have to cut your baby's nails at all at first, as they tend to be very soft. They'll usually just flake off naturally, or you can gently peel away any excess. But once you need to start cutting them, a pair of baby nail scissors or clippers – whichever you feel more comfortable with – will be essential. In my experience, cutting nails while your baby is asleep is your best bet. I know a lot of parents will worry about waking their baby when doing this, but if you wait until she's gone into deep sleep

– in other words, if she's very still and her breathing is slow and regular – you should be fine. I wouldn't even bother trying when she's awake, because she's likely to move and then you risk cutting her. But this way, it doesn't have to be a two-person job.

Aim to follow the shape of the nail, rather than cutting straight across, and don't cut too far down – leave a little of the nail's white tip showing. It's not a good idea to bite or chew nails off, whatever anyone might say. It's too easy to rip off too much.

If you're breastfeeding, you might find you have to trim your baby's toenails, too. I recall getting a scratched tummy when my daughter was being fed with bare feet!

What the netmums say

Getting it nailed

I cut Amelia's nails when she's sleeping, once or twice a week. She'll sleep through anything and this way I don't have to worry about her wriggling. I've got some Tommee Tippee baby nail scissors and baby emery boards, which make it much easier. Someone told me to bite her nails off, but I can't bring myself to bite my own off, let alone my baby's.
Shelley from Swindon, mum to Amelia, four months

Cutting my daughter's nails is a nightmare! They're so sharp and she loves to scratch when she's feeding. It usually takes a good half hour to get them cut as she clenches her fists then gets upset because I won't give her the clippers. I can't do them while she's asleep, because it wakes her up.
Heidi from Warwick, mum to Bella, nine months

I have to cut my boy's nails, as they grow really fast. A friend recommended biting them off, but they're too tiny for my teeth! I was terrified the first time I used clippers and still worry I'm going to draw blood. Now I wait until I'm breastfeeding to do it as that's when he's at his most still. But it can still be tricky.
Clare from Portsmouth, mum to Edward, three months

I always used clippers as I found scissors too scary. I would sit him on my lap and hug him from behind while I sang to him. It must have been a good experience as now he enjoys having them cut, and is even keen to help.
Helen from Cambridge, mum to Adam, four

Whilst cutting my daughter's nails when she was about two months old, I had a terrible experience. I was cutting them with baby nail scissors as my health visitor had showed me, but she started fidgeting and I accidently cut her finger. I was so traumatised by it that I vowed never to cut them again. I still won't. Her father has to do it.
Samantha from Eastbourne, mum to Skye, two

My son has Down's Syndrome, which means he's hypersensitive to touch, so cutting his nails – and hair – has always been potentially traumatic. To this day, I cut them while he's asleep as it causes the least distress, and I tend to just tackle one or two fingers at a time, to minimise the chance of waking him up.
Fran from Bracknell, mum to Harry, three

Ewan is a very wriggly baby and shiny things like scissors seem to attract his attention. As a result, I'm scared that I'll jab him as he tries to lunge at them. I let my mum do it: she seems able to distract and cut at the same time. Nanas are great!
Sian from Glasgow, mum to Ewan, ten months

Several midwives advised me not to bite or cut my son's nails, but to file them instead. I do this when I'm breastfeeding him – with whichever hand is free depending on which boob he's on – or when he's asleep.
Helen from Bristol, mum to Max, six weeks

I use nail clippers and always have. My son hardly slept when he was younger so I did it while he was feeding (with his dad holding the bottle). Now he sits on my knee and I do it when he's calm. After a bath is the best time, when the nails are nice and soft.
Christine from York, mum to Matthew, eleven months

Cutting my little man's nails has always been tricky. He's a real wriggler and now that he always has his hands either clutching something or in his mouth he detests getting interrupted by nail trimming. I tried doing it while he napped but he would just wake up and look at me as though daring me to try. The best method I have found is definitely distraction.

Pam from Arklow, mum to Ruairí, seven months

19 Why do I feel depressed?

If you're unhappy and struggling to cope with life in the months after your baby's birth, it may be that you're suffering from postnatal depression. Statistics vary, but PND is probably more widespread than is often credited: recent research suggests that a staggering one in three women will suffer from it. And PND can happen to women from all walks of life, in any set of circumstances – although some mums are more at risk than others: those with a personal or close family history of depression or other mental health problems, for instance, or those who are under stress anyway for some reason, perhaps because of relationship difficulties or family worries, or if they've been through a difficult previous experience such as miscarriage, birth trauma, domestic violence, or low self-esteem.

Seeking a diagnosis and whatever help you need to overcome PND is vital – for your own sake, for the sake of those around you who love you, and for the sake of your baby, who needs a fully functioning mum to thrive. Your health visitor should be keeping a close eye out for signs of PND and should be your first port of call if you're looking for support. There's also masses of advice to be found on the Netmums website. Prioritise your own emotional wellbeing, if you need to. You can't take care of your baby unless you first take care of yourself.

What the experts say

Crissy says: Whatever you may have heard, postnatal depression is not the same as having the 'baby blues'. The majority of new mums will get the blues to one degree or another soon after giving birth. They may feel tearful, irritable, anxious and sad, but these feelings will generally pass within a few days. Postnatal depression however, typically develops within the first month or two of motherhood – although it may not rear its head for up to a year after your baby is born and for some, symptoms can even develop during pregnancy.

Postnatal depression can be mild, moderate or severe, and can manifest itself in a wide range of often overlapping symptoms. If you're suffering from PND, you may feel frightened, isolated, lonely, confused, angry, anxious, panicky, guilty or ashamed. You may struggle to get to sleep at night or find yourself waking in the early hours, even though you're utterly exhausted and usually can't wait to get to bed. You may be unable to think straight, lose your appetite or seek comfort in eating compulsively, or you may be in despair and unable to cope with things you previously took in your stride. You may feel incapable of caring for your baby and yourself, take little pleasure or interest in your relationships, sex or even your day-to-day life and at times you may just want to hide or run away. You may be tormented by disturbing and distressing thoughts of harming yourself and/or your baby or you may feel sick with worry about your own or your baby's health, his development and safety. There may be physical aches and pains to contend with, such as headaches, stomach pains and a general lack of energy, and you may feel stifled, overwhelmed, and wish you'd never had your baby or feel indifferent or resentful towards him.

I'm not suggesting that any one woman is likely to suffer from all these difficulties, and of course, the severity of each symptom will vary from woman to woman, and also over time. Most women with mild postnatal depression are actually able to function pretty well in their daily lives. Indeed, in its mildest form PND can often go unrecognised and undiagnosed precisely because in a diluted form some of these troubling experiences are actually typical to becoming a mum. However guilty or distressed you may feel, all these thoughts, behaviours and emotions are very common and entirely understand-able for someone suffering from postnatal depression. The crucial point here is that if you experience five or more of these symptoms, continuing over a period of two weeks or more, you need to seek help. If in doubt or if someone close to you is concerned for your welfare but you think you're fine, please seek help anyway. Don't assume that if you push your feelings aside and carry on regardless things will spontaneously improve. The chances are they probably won't, so is it really worth taking the risk? When mums suffer from postnatal depression they often fear being judged by others, but ironically, they are generally their own worst critics. Being unable to pull themselves together and shake off their depression can leave them feeling inadequate, which isn't helped if, having reached rock bottom themselves, they end up comparing themselves unfavourably to other mums who may on the surface appear to be sailing through motherhood in a rose-tinted haze.

In the first instance it really doesn't matter who you reach out to: the most important thing is that you find someone to talk to whom you can trust. If you don't know your midwife or health visitor that well, call your GP, and if you can't face talking to a health professional at all, try opening up to your partner, friend or a family member and enlisting their support in taking the next step. And remember, even in your darkest moments, that your situation is far from hopeless. PND can be overcome and there are a range of treatment options available for you including medication, counsel-ling, psychotherapy or group therapies, online and face-to-face PND support networks and holistic or homeopathic remedies.

What the netmums say

Beyond the 'baby blues'

My first pregnancy was going well and I felt fantastic, but at thirty-six weeks they found the baby's heart rate was high. I was sent to hospital, and Ella was born by emergency C-section. As her lungs were not developed enough she spent a week in SCBU. I felt the care I received in the hospital was poor and there was no explan-ation as to why things happened as they did. I know it sounds daft, but I just wasn't prepared for a baby a few weeks early. I never expected to have a C-section, and not to be able to hold or feed my baby. At home, I just felt that I could not cope. She was such a good girl but it was just too much for me. I panicked all the time about her dying, and cried at everything. My stepfather found a PND support group where we lived and they were fantastic, ringing, emailing and just making sure I was OK for a long time after. My partner was amazing, my rock. I do not know how he coped with me and a new baby. He says that he had to believe that life would get back to how it used to be.

I was an only child myself and did not want a lonely childhood for Ella, so we made a decision to try for a second baby. Kill or cure. The pregnancy was stressful and then, at twenty-nine weeks, I saw a different consultant and she finally explained why they had to deliver Ella the way they had. It was like something clicked. I wish I'd been told this at the time. When Grace was born, I was able to feed her and change her nappy as a new mum should. I felt bad about my feelings towards Ella but know it was not my fault, or hers, or her sister's. The anxiety still rears its head sometimes, when I get stressed or over-tired, and especially when Ella is ill. Her dad has to deal with it, as I just freak out. I also struggle in the run-up to her birthday, but I just get on with it, bake a cake, and find a corner to cry in. I have taken each day at a time, and tried not to push myself. Over time, I've learned to love Ella and love being with her, which at times I thought would never happen.
Louise from Sheffield, mum to Ella, two, and Grace, six months

I had PND with my first daughter, Abigail. I had a really bad pregnancy and think I probably slipped into depression even before the birth. Because I suffered from SPD, a disabling pregnancy-related condition, I had to have a planned C-section and afterwards I felt completely numb. Although I knew I loved my baby, I just did not connect with her. I was severely anaemic after the section and then had a bad skin reaction to the iron medication I had to take. My SPD still meant I was not very mobile, and my days blended into each other just sat in the house caring for my baby. I think she was about eight weeks old when I knew I was not right. Luckily my GP was fantastic and offered both antidepressants and cognitive behaviour therapy (CBT). Apparently I had the type of PND where you can care for your baby and move through life, but without actually feeling part of it. I did not feel constantly upset; I just did not seem to have any feelings about anything – good or bad. The worst parts were the side effects: always feeling tired, having anxiety attacks, paranoia that 'they' would take my baby away. It seems ridiculous when I look back now, especially as I had a supportive husband and family. For the CBT, a counsellor came to my house and it made a world of difference being able to offload my worries and find solutions for what I saw as problems. I went back to work part-time when she was six months old and I really believed this helped me immensely. I came off the antidepressants and in 2009 we decided to try for another baby. I knew there was a good chance of the PND returning but the pregnancy could not have been more different. This time, the bond was there from the start. It does make me feel like I missed out on things the first time round, but I love both my children to bits and am just relieved that PND is something you *can* recover from – even though it does not seem like it at the time.

Stephanie from Barnsley, mum to Abigail, seven, and Olivia, eighteen months

My PND has been a long journey, and honestly it's not over, although every day I wish (and sometimes pretend) I have overcome it. I am a strong, independent woman who was really ready to have a family, and I have an equally strong and supportive husband. My little girl eats well, smiles and laughs easily, and was sleeping through the night from six weeks, so from the outside, everything looked perfect. I'm good at masking my true feelings to others and was so certain the numbness I felt, the constant anxiety, and not feeling like I was cut out for it all was just a normal part of being a new mum. People would say things like, 'Oh, they grow so fast, enjoy every minute of it,' and it would fill me with dread and despair.

When my girl was about eight weeks old, I shared a few of my feelings with a couple of fellow mums, thinking it was small talk. Their reactions made it clear that what I was feeling was not normal. I

took a PND test that I found on Netmums and my score was scarily high. Even after that it took my husband driving me to the doctor's office and waiting outside with my daughter for me to actually get help. I told my health visitor as well. I began taking anti-depressants and had several free counselling sessions through a charity. I felt like I was lifted out of a fog when the medication finally kicked in and for the most part I've been back to myself for several months now. I still feel guilty for not recognising it sooner and when I'm stressed, I drop so much lower than I ever did before. When I think of someone with a newborn, I automatically feel sad and worried for them. I get tearful whenever I think about missing the first several months of my little girl's life. However, I'm so glad I got help. It was such a relief when I realised it wasn't just me and I didn't bring it on myself! It's a shame that the stigma surrounding PND makes it a taboo subject. I was determined to be open and honest about it once I recovered and yet I worry about any colleagues knowing I suffered. I wish I'd known to get help sooner but I am so grateful for those who shared their stories with me. I hope my story can help someone else, if nothing else than by letting them know they are not alone.
Sandy from Bristol, mum to Molly, fifteen months

I believe I'm currently suffering with PND. I've made a few unsuccessful attempts to make a doctor's appointment, and have given up trying for now whilst I build my courage back up. Whilst I was pregnant I was so excited, I couldn't wait to meet my daughter. The pregnancy went smoothly, but the birth was overdue, with a long labour and complications. However, I felt fine in the early weeks. I was so happy she'd arrived and I could finally enjoy her. Within a month, though, I was being plagued by horrible thoughts, convinced someone was going to take her from me. One night I cried for ages because I couldn't find her, until I remembered she was sleeping with her nan that night. From then on my paranoia got worse. I wouldn't go out because I was scared that someone would take her, or hurt her, or she would get hit by a car or a bus. I kept feeling so bad I didn't want to wake in the morning and at one point I thought of putting her up for adoption because I wasn't the mother she needed. It got worse when my aunt dropped her one day. She was fine but I felt awful, as though I hadn't done

enough to protect her. I even began thinking about self-harm, and suicide. I still suffer anxiety and panic attacks every time our doorbell goes. But I'm planning to pull through this for her and be the mummy she needs, and I want to beat it alone. Right now it feels like a long shot, but I know I won't always be like this. She needs a working mummy, not a broken one.
Lara from Stafford, mum to Betsy, six months

My then partner and I were over the moon when we found out I was pregnant again. Pregnancy, birth and breastfeeding all seemed to go pretty well. We were all very happy, or so I thought. My son became very ill at five weeks and had to go back to hospital for three days, to be fed by a tube, which was distressing, but he recovered and we went home. Then I found out that my other half had been having an affair with someone from work, and had been suspended. He'd slept with her the night I was in hospital, giving birth to our son. My entire world came crashing down around me. It felt like someone had ripped the carpet from under my feet. The next few months went by in a blur. I was forced to return to work when my son was only ten weeks old, as my other half was not earning. Working sixty-hour weeks took a serious toll on me, and my relationship with my son particularly. Stupidly I stuck with my other half, but the relationship was damaged beyond repair and that was having a knock-on effect for my son. It was awful. I couldn't be around him on my own for any length of time as I would panic and couldn't look after him. I couldn't cope with his crying. I completely ignored him at times and barely had any contact with him. I went on feeling like this for probably four months before I spoke to anyone about it. I felt so ashamed that I didn't love my poor little boy. I finally relented and spoke to my health visitor, giving her the full background story. It was like a huge weight was lifted off my shoulders. She told me what I was feeling was OK and that in time my son and I would get our relationship back on track. She came to our house for home visits and reassured me so much that I could do it and I would get there with him. I am still recovering now, and we have good days and bad days. As a result of my neglect, he is a very needy little boy. I do love him dearly and things are looking much brighter, especially as my ex now lives 500 miles away. It's not easy trying to

cope alone with two demanding little ones, but I'm taking it step by step and you know what? I wouldn't have it any other way.
Hollie from Weymouth, mum to Millie, three, and Mason, fourteen months

I think I suffered from undiagnosed PND. It was a difficult birth, with several complications. And once home, I was a bit shell-shocked as the reality of my new life kicked in. Joey was a poor sleeper from the start. He hardly napped, aside from the odd snatched half hour, so the advice to 'sleep when your baby sleeps' felt like a slap in the face. Night times were not much better. I was exhausted even before he was born, and suffered from such broken sleep I was a walking zombie. I often felt light-headed and dizzy and was afraid of falling down the stairs. I also experienced night sweats in the first week or so and would wake up several times in the night, soaking wet and freezing. Joey was breastfeeding and an enormous eater, so perhaps I wasn't eating or drinking enough in the early weeks. Physically, my recovery was slow: my stitches took a very long time to heal, and an anal fissure meant excruciating pain every time I opened my bowels. I did try to get out with Joey regularly, but it was difficult as I was so exhausted. I don't have a large support network, and I figured that as my husband was the one working and bringing home the pay, my job was to look after Joey and the house, so I didn't ask for help from him – which was a big mistake. Most of the time, I felt an enormous sense of anxiety and frequently struggled to cope. This has only just changed. I feel as though I have come through the tunnel and now know the joy of motherhood. And how sweet it is!
Anna from Birmingham, mum to Joey, three

To be honest, the early days are a complete blur. I was bedbound for twenty-four hours after the birth and really struggled with breast-feeding. Night feeds were the worst: when I think about that time now it seems like a dream. I feel like PND settled in without me even noticing it. It wasn't until I was quite bad, after about three months, that I thought something was wrong, but I turned a blind eye and didn't get help. Neither my husband or health visitor seemed to recognise it, so I suffered in silence thinking it would pass. It made the first year of my daughter's life very hard for me. I put a lot of

pressure on myself and put a 'brave face' on for the outside world. I still managed to bond with her and enjoy local activities with her at the children's centres and I still feel very protective of her. Two years on, I'm a lot better, but still recovering.
Jenny from Stockport, mum to Laila, two

Before I had my third child, I didn't understand PND at all. I've got to be honest and say that if anyone told me they had it, I'd say, 'Yes, a baby changes your life and it's hard – but get over it!' It wasn't until after my third birth that I fully understood what PND is all about. My pregnancy had been a breeze (as had all my pregnancies) but my son became distressed during labour and he was born by C-section, for which I had a general anaesthetic. For the first few months after his birth, I felt the usual euphoria, but by about four months I felt incredibly low. Things slowly got worse and worse until my mum said she thought I had PND. It was like a light had been switched on for me. I understood why I'd been having suicidal thoughts. I'd be driving along and would suddenly just think to myself, I could just drive into that wall and be done with it, kill us all, the world is such a dreadful place. I felt like I'd be saving my children from something terrible. My PND lasted for about two years. Not all of it was to the point of contemplating suicide, but it was like having a huge weight on my shoulders that just wouldn't go away. I felt guilty and stupid that before this time I had completely dismissed women with PND as 'pathetic'.
Michelle from Blandford, mum to Ruby, ten, Anna, six, and Toby, four

Harry was a planned baby, who I was very excited about – particularly as I'd suffered three previous miscarriages. Unfortunately I wasn't diagnosed with PND until ten months after Harry's birth, and I still don't remember parts of my life, or Harry's, from that time, which makes me feel bad even now. I don't remember washing, eating, showering, going to loo, or doing any housework. I do remember trying to go out to the shops, and being terrified that he might cry and that I wouldn't know what to do, and then everyone would be looking at me and judging me and thinking I was a bad mum. My mood swings at home were awful too. I would easily go from being OK to being really angry and upset, then to feeling completely despairing of everything. I would get visions of things happening, such as falling down the stairs with Harry, and him ending up getting hurt, so I would have to go to hospital, and then he'd be taken away from me. I got help from my lovely GP, who prescribed me with anti-depressants, and referred me to the mental health team. I ended up working with an absolutely fantastic charity, which, along with their partnership with CBT therapists, helped save me. It took six months to get my medication right, and in that time I can honestly say I would not have coped without that charity. I was further beyond any despair I'd ever experienced before (and I suffered from depression when I was younger), and felt so down I regularly wondered why I was bothering at all and whether there was going to be an end to it all. Then my GP changed my medication, and it was like a veil I'd been wearing was finally being lifted. I was able to spend time with relatives or close friends (something I'd been reluctant to do before that) and even take Harry out. I decided to leave my job as it was rather stressful, and probably not helping my situation, particularly as my boss was far from understanding. Now, although I still have days where I feel despondent, I know how to deal with it. I think, 'OK, bad day today, let's start again tomorrow.' I even know how to try and avoid feeling like that. With me, it's making sure I have something planned for each day of the week, even if it's just 'tackle the kitchen and then go and do some shopping'. And I have to say I'm extremely proud when I think of how far I've travelled. I'm now in the process of reducing my meds, and am looking to the future. I would like to try for another baby maybe towards the end of the year, and am in the very early stages of setting up my own business. Although I hated the way PND made me feel and think, part of me is glad I've had it. I'm a stronger person who's come out the other side of something awful, and it's made me the person I am today.

Melanie from Kingshurst, mum to Harry, two

20 What should I do about cradle cap?

Cradle cap is a scaly, yellow, greasy covering of the scalp that very commonly appears in young babies in the first three months and can hang around for quite a while, occasionally into toddlerhood. Your baby is unlikely to be bothered by it, but you might be, because severe cases can look pretty unpleasant. It can build up to quite a thick crust, so if you're going to attempt to get rid of it, it's probably better to try sooner rather than later.

Confusingly, there seems to be a lot of potential remedies out there, with some mums swearing by methods that others have found useless. You may just have to try several different approaches to see which works best – steering clear, of course, of anything that could be harmful and halting immediately if anything seems to irritate or worsen it. Many mums struggle to resist temptation when it comes to picking at cradle cap, as the scales can seem so . . . well, pickable. But it's something to avoid, because it could make the area vulnerable to infection. If you're not bothered too much by the way it looks, and your baby doesn't seem to care either, an option is simply to leave cradle cap and wait for it to go of its own accord, which it will eventually. And in the meantime, of course, there are always hats!

What the experts say

Maggie says: Doctors can't agree totally on a cause for cradle cap, but it's definitely not a lack of hygiene and it's extremely common, so you don't have to feel bad if your baby has it. It's a form of skin condition called seborrhoeic dermatitis and the most likely theory is that it's a result of overactive sebaceous (oil producing) glands, ramped up by hormones passed on by the mum during pregnancy. The excess sebum (or oil) causes old skin cells to stick to the scalp, rather than fall off as they usually do.

There are many old wives' tales and anecdotal 'cures' for cradle cap and very little in the way of medical evidence or official guidelines, so it's hard to advise on it definitively. All you can do really is pick one method and give it a go. There are a number of suitable emollient creams which you can either get over the counter – ask the pharmacist first to make sure it's suitable – or have prescribed by your GP. Otherwise a natural oil such as olive oil or baby oil, or petroleum jelly can have the same effect – but bear in mind all these things can leave the hair and head very greasy, and are sometimes hard to wash out completely. Do also avoid nut-based oils, because of the risk of an allergic reaction. After washing, you should be able to lift off flakes using a soft brush. I've never tried it myself, but another safe home remedy said to work is a paste of water and bicarbonate of soda, left on for ten minutes before washing it off. Stick to a mild shampoo – or you could try a medicated variety such as Dentinox, which is specially formulated for cradle cap and recommended by many parents.

There's no doubt that a bad case of cradle cap can look really horrible, especially if it spreads down to the eyes and eyebrows as it sometimes does, and I can see why so many mums want to get rid of it. The problem is that even if you remove it, it will usually come back. If you don't bother to try and treat it, it will go eventually – although it's possible it will be an issue for up to two years, and in a few cases, beyond. There may be consolation in the fact that once your baby has a good head of hair, it won't be so noticeable.

Dr David says: Many parents feel cradle cap is just something they have to put up with, but it can look really nasty. So if you're concerned, see your doctor who can prescribe a suitable mois-turising cream to use on it – or you can get one over the counter, asking the pharmacist's advice first. If it's really persistent, or if it's causing any itching or discomfort to your baby, or seems red and inflamed, it may be that either a fungal infection or eczema has developed, and you should definitely get it checked out. Picking at it can definitely increase the risk of infection . . . so try not to!

What the netmums say

Tackling cradle cap

Danny had, and still has to an extent, cradle cap. It's never been really awful but his hair is blond and quite fine so occasionally it has been quite noticeable. It's never bothered him though and because of that it's never really bothered me. However, my sister very tactfully once described his flaky scalp as 'minging', which made me think it might be noticeable to other people. As it was itchy, I never put anything on it. Some people suggested massaging olive oil into his scalp but the thought of cleaning that out of his bed sheets put me off. As he has got older and his hair has got thicker, it's got a lot better.
Cathy from Reading, mum to Danny, two

Both mine had cradle cap, even in their eyebrows. I found putting baby oil on their head then going through with a plastic nit comb worked better than any of the special shampoos I tried.
Charlotte from Burnley, mum to Daisy, three, and Mia, eight months

My wee boy got dreadful cradle cap all over his scalp at around eight weeks. I was advised to rub in olive oil initially but it didn't help – if anything it seemed to dry his cradle cap out. A different GP recommended Dentinox shampoo and combing his hair after application, making sure not to pick at flakes and to keep an eye on them in case they became infected. I bathed him every night while it persisted and combed through the hair, and it was gone within a week.
Ruth from Dumbarton, mum to Robbie, two, and Anna, one month

I tried olive oil on my daughter's cradle cap, but it made her smell like an old chip pan so I didn't persist after the first application.

Someone then recommended aqueous cream, so I bought some from Boots and gave it a whirl. It worked a treat.
Miranda from Hertford, mum to Mimi, two

Both my daughters had terrible cradle cap. We used olive oil with both which worked . . . eventually. But with my second, someone suggested Vaseline, and I'm not exaggerating when I say I covered her head with it overnight and by the morning once I had brushed it out it was all gone! It was one of the best tips I was ever given as a new mum.
Julia from Harrow, mum to Martha, three, and Tess, six months

Both my girls had cradle cap, and I left it to work its own way off. My health visitor was most surprised by this and claimed it would never come off by itself, but it did . . . although with my first daughter I admit I helped it along a little by picking bits off!
Charlotte from Morpeth, mum to Leah, three, and Rebekah, nineteen months

Head & Shoulders does the trick! My daughter started getting cradle cap at around three weeks of age and I remembered hearing a friend recommend a mild anti-dandruff shampoo. I started using a tiny amount a couple of times a week and within two weeks it had already started clearing. It's now nearly gone.
Louise from Poole, mum to Leanna, two months

My son had cradle cap and it looked awful. I tried putting olive oil on it overnight and gently brushing the flakes out – until he developed a rash on his face that dried up and got quite sore. I tried aqueous cream, and something called Diprobase that the GP prescribed, and neither worked. In the end, the thing that cleared up both the rash and the cradle cap was Oilatum, a bath emollient.
Jessica from Bristol, mum to Marley, two

William had a lot of hair so his awful case of cradle cap was a bit of a nightmare! We found the best solution to be an emollient cream called Epaderm. We just rubbed a good whack on forty-five

minutes before bath time then brushed it through, washed his hair, then ran a comb through in a zigzag to lift the flakes gently, and washed it again. After two nights, it was gone. When it returned a while later my mum tried putting Vaseline in his hair but it just wouldn't come out and he ended up with a haircut. As for picking, I just managed to refrain – but it took almost chopping my fingers off!
Marianne from Uddingston, mum to William, twenty-two months

My daughter used to get cradle cap. I used Dentinox shampoo (and yes, I picked!). I found that washing her hair too often seemed to be the problem – so now I only wash it when it needs it and she doesn't get it any more.
Kirsty from Musselburgh, mum to Ellie, four

I left E45 cream on my son's head overnight then used a nit comb to take the flakes off in the morning. He hasn't had it since.
Leighann from Manchester, mum to Zack, six, and Kane, two

My son had it pretty badly from three months, for about six weeks. We tried olive oil and a few other home remedies before taking him to the doctor, who prescribed Epaderm emollient to use as a shampoo, and Oilatum cream to rub on afterwards. By the morning, most of the flakes were on his bed sheet and after a fortnight, they were completely gone. I did pick it at the beginning, but I think I actually made it worse and my partner told me off, so I stopped!
Abigail from Bristol, mum to Frank, six months

PART THREE: 3–6 MONTHS

21 When will he sleep through?

Sleep deprivation can be torture. It's one of the hardest things about having a new baby. Not surprisingly, new parents want to know when they can start looking forward to a whole night's sleep again. And other parents will probably want to know your sleeping status, too. 'Is he going through the night yet?' is the question you're most likely to hear at mum and baby groups.

Fact is, young babies wake at night – sometimes once, sometimes repeatedly. In the early months, their tummies are still small and need regular refills (even at antisocial hours!) and their body clocks have yet to settle into what the rest of us see as a normal pattern. It's impossible to say when *your* baby will sleep through the night, as all babies are different. If you're unusually lucky, he may do so of his own accord, from six to eight weeks. But most babies will carry on waking at least once a night far beyond that. Once he's six months old and well established on solids, it's usually possible to 'teach' a baby how to sleep through, if that's a route you want to go down. (For more on sleep training, see Question 35.) In the meantime, you can help him develop good sleeping habits that will pave the way to a good night's sleep, eventually – for everyone.

What the experts say

Maggie says: As a newborn, your baby will have very erratic sleeping habits, partly because his circadian rhythm, or body clock, has yet to develop, and partly because the size of his tummy means he'll want small but very regular feeds – so he's likely to wake several times in the night needing a top-up, or maybe even just a cuddle. It's a case of gritting your teeth and bearing it at this stage because babies this young must be given whatever they need to make them happy. The flipside is that they also sleep in the day so hopefully you can catch up on a bit of kip then.

As time goes on, he'll spend more time awake in the day, and wake less frequently at night. Lots of parents find that three months is a bit of a turning point, in particular, because by then the body clock has regulated, and levels of melatonin, the sleep hormone, have increased. He'll be able to take bigger feeds, and will naturally be able to go for longer stretches in between. However, at this stage, one or two night wakings are still normal, and you may have a while to go before you can say that he's 'sleeping through' – although interestingly, health professionals usually define sleeping through as a stretch of unbroken sleep lasting six hours or more, so perhaps your baby is doing better than you realise.

Some mums are happy to let nature – and their baby – lead the way when it comes to sleeping through. But many of us become too desperate for that, and want to know how we can speed up the process. The good news is that, although it's not advisable to launch a committed programme of sleep training with a baby of less than six months, you can still set up some early habits that will really help if it's a good night's sleep you're after. For instance, you can help your baby – from day one – to understand the difference between day and night, which will help those circadian rhythms slot into place. So, aim to keep lights low and eye contact and chat to a minimum when feeding or changing him at night, whereas in the daytime, make sure the curtains are drawn back, and spend his waking times chatting and playing. Getting him out and about in the daylight is a good idea – as well as aiding the development of the body clock, it can boost production of melatonin.

The other really vital step you can take is teaching your baby to 'self-settle'. That means putting him down to sleep awake and leaving him to drop off on his own. This may be easier said than done with a newborn, who will often cry and want to be soothed, rocked or fed to sleep, but nevertheless, it's a good idea to start encouraging your baby to self-settle as early as possible, because what you're aiming for is for him to get himself back to sleep when he wakes in the night, rather than waking you and demanding your services. It's key to getting a good night's sleep!

Up until he's six months, it's not fair to deny a baby night-time feeds if he seems to want them, as he could genuinely be waking from hunger. But you can aim to 'space them out' a bit, after about three months, by which time most babies shouldn't need more than one or two feeds to get them through the night. Aim to increase the space in between feeds by short periods of fifteen minutes or so by making him wait a while rather than jumping up to attend to him, and then perhaps distracting him with a stroke or a cuddle. After a few nights of this spacing process you should find your baby's waking schedule has adjusted accordingly, and then you can aim to extend the gap by a further fifteen minutes, and so on.

Some parents find that offering a 'dream feed' – in other words, waking their sleeping baby for a feed, just before their own bedtime, buys them a more prolonged stretch of sleep than they would otherwise get. Personally, I'd advise against this, as it can interfere with a baby's natural sleep/wake rhythm, and I'm not convinced it will definitely have the desired effect! But there's probably no harm in trying dream feeding and, if you find it works for you, you could stick with it until your baby is able to get through the night without it, and then you can simply drop it.

Finally, whether or not you are the sort of parent who prefers to run your baby's life to a strict schedule, establishing a bedtime routine is an all-important move. It's a good idea to do this early, although most parents find there's not a lot of point trying much before six weeks, when their baby's sleeping and feeding patterns are so erratic. (For more on bedtime routines, see Question 16.)

Lots of breastfeeding mums wonder if a bottle of formula given last thing at night will help. In fact, research suggests that breastfed babies are usually only a few short weeks behind when it comes to 'sleeping through', but it's true that formula isn't digested as easily as breast milk and is likely to leave a baby feeling fuller for longer. If you're truly exhausted, it may be worth trying. Do be aware that your milk production will reduce accordingly if you take this route – and also that breastfeeding at night is said to have particularly beneficial effects, as naturally occurring chemicals that are linked to sleepiness, called nucleotides, only reach their highest concentration in breast milk that's produced at night. Starting solids can *sometimes* have the effect of improving sleep at night – however, that's no reason to begin weaning earlier than recommended (for more on when to wean, see Question 30). It's definitely a bad idea to add cereal or extra formula to his milk feeds in the hope of buying yourself some more sleep because not only is that a choking risk, it could cause him to become constipated or dehydrated.

Crissy says: Don't be taken in by those experienced veteran mums or seemingly perfect rookies whose rose-coloured recollections or apparently super-human feats of stamina may fool you into thinking that you too should be able to push through the exhaustion barrier and carry on regardless. The truth of the matter is that we humans need sleep and when we don't get it we feel pretty rubbish. Sleep deprivation can lower your mood, leaving you feeling overwhelmed, weepy, irritable, and constantly on a short fuse. It may also affect your physical health, leaving you more prone to minor illnesses, or impact on your cognitive ability until you find yourself quite literally unable to think straight. Over time, a chronic lack of sleep can even make you more susceptible to depression, panic and anxiety.

But while there's no doubt that sleep deprivation can bring the most capable mother to her knees, what often troubles a new mum even more is the belief that her baby's night waking is somehow her fault. When you have unrealistically high expectations of yourself and your baby, chances are at some point you'll both fall short of the mark. Every baby is different and just like walking and talking, sleeping through the night is a developmental milestone that your baby will reach in his own sweet time. If you're feeling that you don't measure up to other mothers, remember that those super-competitive mums at baby group were almost certainly every bit as competitive before Junior came along, so you can guarantee that once they've got sleeping firmly under their belt their kids will quickly graduate to eating solids, potty training and composing symphonies, so it's pretty much always going to be a no-win situation for us mere mortals. Oh, and don't forget: you've only got their word for it that their little darlings have been slumbering all night from a mere six weeks!

What the netmums say

Sleeping like a baby

In the first weeks, my eldest used to wake up every three hours for a feed. He quickly started sleeping longer stretches and by six weeks he slept from 11 p.m. until 6 a.m. By the time he was four months old he was sleeping fourteen hours non-stop – although he tended to be awake a lot during the day so I guess it was just catching up. My youngest used to wake at least every two hours for feeds and did so for a long time. I was absolutely shattered! It did improve, but it wasn't until he turned six months that he finally slept through.
Irma from Oldham, mum to Damir, four, and Aydin, two

I was lucky with my son: he put himself in a routine after the first couple of days and would wake every four hours for a feed. He started sleeping through at six weeks and since then we've had only one broken night's sleep. Fingers crossed that baby number two will follow in her brother's footsteps!
Laura from Preston, mum to Joel, two

What is this sleep of which you speak? I'm still waiting on sleeping through, but I know she will in her own time. It doesn't stop others hinting that if I give her a bottle of formula she would sleep better. I am happy to breastfeed her at night, thanks.
Amanda from Fleet, mum to Tabitha, nine months

At twelve weeks, my boys go down at 7.30 p.m. Jack will then wake at half four, and Rylan at half five, and they'll both have a bottle of formula before going back to sleep until 8 a.m. I have always formula fed, on demand, and up until about eight or nine

weeks they fed every two and a half to three hours, even through the night. I kept on putting them to bed at the same time, and kept all feeds after that until 6 a.m. as 'night feeds' – lights dim, minimal interaction, feed, burp, quick change, and put back in cot whether awake or asleep. I also found that they always need a good nap after their midday feed for this to work best. I don't want to jinx myself but, so far, so good.
Rosie from Antrim, mum to Jack and Rylan, four months

My boys did not start to sleep through until they were eighteen months old. Incidentally, this was also the age when they decided not to breastfeed any more. I was quite happy with both things. I was asked by the health visitor to go to a sleep clinic after I told her that they didn't sleep through at twelve months, but as I wasn't concerned by the situation I turned her down. I was happy to allow them to do it all in their own time. I was tired, especially when they woke four or five times in the night, but on the whole it was liveable with as it was my choice!
Ruth from Rugby, mum to Gregory, eight, and Nicholas, six

Our fourth daughter still isn't sleeping through the night. She wakes every two to three hours for a comfort feed and because there are other children in the house who are at school and also need to sleep, I pander to her. I'm one very tired momma!
Rachel from Southampton, mum to Farhanna, eleven, Amber, ten, Zaara, four, and Amelia, eleven months

Kobey has been sleeping well since he was about six months old, usually from about 7.30 p.m. to 6.30 a.m. It happened after he had been ill with a cold; something seemed to change after that and he no longer needed a night feed. It also coincided with the introduction of solids into his diet, so it may be that he was nice and full during the day. He is yet to teethe though – so I am enjoying it whilst I can!
Janine from Caerphilly, mum to Kobey, eight months

My little girl first slept from 7 p.m. to 7 a.m. on Christmas Eve, when she was just short of nine months – a lovely present for mummy!

Before that she would always wake once, at 11 p.m. My health visitor had advised me to just give her water if she woke as she was capable of going through, and it may have just been habit. Since then she has had the odd night of waking if teething or poorly, but is now a pretty good sleeper.
Julie from Peterborough, mum to Trinity, fifteen months

Bethany is still not sleeping through. She manages 7 p.m. to 4.30 a.m. but can't seem to get past the 4.30 a.m. feed, although she only drinks about 3 fl oz and then goes straight back down until 7 a.m. I have tried not giving her milk when she wakes, but she won't settle without it. I must admit, I get fed up with other mums telling me she should be sleeping through by now. All babies are different, and she'll do it in her own time.
Victoria from St Albans, mum to Bethany, seven months

My son slept through from two months old. He was bottle-fed, and always had a good appetite. At the opposite end of the spectrum, we're still waiting for my daughter to sleep through and she's ten months old. She's never really drunk masses of milk. She usually sleeps from 7 p.m. till 10 p.m., and can then be awake until 1 a.m. People suggest we try controlled crying, but we're worried it would wake her brother up. It's a no-win situation!
Karen from Warrington, mum to Matthew, two, and Katie, ten months

Elliot slept through at five weeks, from 10.30 p.m. to 6 a.m. He was breastfed and swaddled – I'm not sure if that made a difference, or not. The only time we have disturbed nights now is when he's ill, which thankfully isn't very often.
Jeni-Ann from Darwen, mum to Elliot, two

As a newborn, my daughter only ever woke once during the night. We'd put her down at 10 p.m., she would wake for a feed at about 3 a.m., and then she slept until 7 a.m. However, at eight weeks she started sleeping through entirely.
Fiona from Alfreton, mum to Miread, four

We had a bedtime routine from day one – bath, sleep suit on, bottle, story, and into the cot awake – which I think really worked for us. We'd always get her dressed for the day first thing in the morning, and I think that helped establish a difference between day and night. At three weeks she started sleeping through completely, having previously been put to bed at 8 p.m., given a 'dream feed' at midnight, then waking up for a bottle at 4 a.m. and being awake for the day at 8 a.m. At five weeks she dropped the dream feed, too.

Caroline from Manchester, mum to Natalia, ten months

Isobel slept from 10 p.m. to 6 a.m. from about fourteen weeks until eighteen weeks, then started waking again. People said we should wean to get her sleeping again, but I wanted to wait. She settled back to sleeping from 10 p.m. to 3 a.m. within a couple of weeks, and is gradually extending this now, with occasional nights of waking more regularly. I have no intention of sleep training. We co-sleep, and will do for as long as she needs me.

Claire from Southampton, mum to Isobel, seven months

22 How can I introduce a bottle?

Many breastfeeding mums reach a point where they want to offer one or more feeds from a bottle, rather than the boob. Whether you're sticking with your own milk, expressed, or you're switching in part or entirely to formula, you'll need to find a way to interest your baby in this new way of feeding, and it may not be a simple swap. Bottle teats are not as soft as nipples, and she may object to being offered silicone rather than skin. She may also initially find the change of taste disagreeable, if you're offering formula for the first time, in place of breast milk. For this reason, it's a good idea, if you know you will want a bottle to be an option at some stage, to offer one fairly early on. Six to eight weeks is reckoned to be an ideal window of opportunity – in other words, after breastfeeding has had a good chance to get established, but before your baby becomes so accustomed to the boob that she simply won't countenance an alternative. Of course, you may not feel ready to offer anything other than the breast to your baby at that stage. Just be aware that it can be harder the longer you put it off. In fact, some mums find that there's just no interesting their baby in a bottle, however hard they try!

Don't neglect the importance of hygiene when you're offering milk in a bottle. Always wash bottles and teats and breast pumps thoroughly in very hot, soapy water, and sterilise daily in a steam or microwave steriliser, or by using sterilising solution. (Breast pumps, nipple shields, dummies and teething toys should also be sterilised regularly too.) The various sterilising methods have their pros and cons, depending on whether price, convenience or capacity is your priority, but they all work equally well as long as you follow the instructions carefully. Be sure, too, to make up formula feeds exactly as directed on the tin. (There's more about sterilising, and when it's OK to stop, in Question 34.)

What the experts say

Maggie says: I think it's a good idea for all babies – even those that are exclusively breastfed – to be happy about taking a bottle. For that reason, I've always advised breastfeeding mums to offer supplementary drinks of water in a bottle from quite an early stage (although, assuming you're keen to carry on with at least some breastfeeding, I'd recommend waiting for four to six weeks before offering a bottle, so that your baby doesn't become confused by being offered both). That way, if you get stuck somewhere and you're not around to feed your baby when she needs it, at least someone can offer her a drink of water – or even, if it came to it, a bottle of formula. It will also make life a lot easier if and when you want to introduce a bottle more regularly, or make a perma-nent switch. And mixing bottle and breastfeeding *can* work very well, in spite of the common view that it's a 'slippery slope' that will soon bring about a complete end to breastfeeding. Mums who return to work, for instance, often find a good compromise in leaving a bottle for their baby during the day, whilst still offering a breastfeed in the morning and/or at night.

There are various tricks to try when you're attempting to intro-duce your baby to the bottle. Making sure the milk's at the right temperature can help – if it's formula, and you want it to taste as close to your breast milk as you can, it should be slightly warm. It might also be necessary to get the timing right – the best window is probably when your baby is hungry, but not over-hungry, which could mean she's already distressed and therefore not in a very receptive mood.

If you're not getting anywhere, it's a good idea to ask someone who isn't breastfeeding to do the honours, because if your baby smells your milk that's bound to make it harder. It might also be worth trying a different type of teat – they come with varying rates of flows, and in different materials and shapes, so you might need to offer several before hitting on one your baby will go for. For instance, you might find a teat made of latex to be more appealing than silicone, as it's softer and more nipple-like.

When it comes to introducing a bottle, you may need to keep persevering for quite a while. Try to take a relaxed approach, if possible – it's a good idea to wait a couple of days in between attempts. If you need to get your baby taking a bottle for a particular reason – that return to work, for instance – make sure you've got plenty of time to achieve success.

Failing everything else, there's always the 'cold turkey' approach, based on the theory that your baby will *have* to accept a bottle if she becomes hungry enough. Be warned though, they can hold out for a long time: you may find your nerves desert you, and that you give in before she does. You might be better off asking someone else to do this for you – if you can find someone willing to go through with it.

A lot of breastfed babies just will *not* drink from a bottle, full stop. If you're struggling, you might find she will drink expressed or formula milk from a 'Doidy cup' or sippy cup, instead, from six months or so. But on the other hand, you might just decide you don't need the hassle and continue offering nothing but the breast indefinitely. I do sympathise with this problem, as none of my babies would accept a changeover to the bottle in spite of my efforts – although I recall that I managed to convince one of them to suck from a straw, which was something at least!

What the netmums say

Hitting the bottle

I am trying desperately to do this now! My daughter has always refused a bottle, whether it contains formula, expressed breastmilk, water or juice. She won't accept milk in a sippy cup either, she just clamps her lips shut, although she will happily drink water from one. I've tried distraction, asking somebody else to give it to her, offering it when she's half asleep, and at different times of the day – when she's starving, when she's just peckish, when she's not hungry at all! And I've spent a fortune on different bottles, beakers, and teats. She's such a happy baby I am loath to go cold turkey as I can't bear the thought of her screaming it out, but I'm thinking that it might be the only way.

Laura from London, mum to Nicholas, two, and Eloise, eight months

I had to switch my daughter to bottle-feeds a couple of weeks ago. She was admitted to hospital with severe reflux and they wanted to see if changing her feed would help. It was a complete nightmare, with staff and my husband trying to get her to take hypoallergenic formula in a hospital bottle. Eventually they let me express some milk and my husband managed to get her to take some. I went home from hospital really worried as I knew that she would need feeding overnight – the nurses planned to tube feed her if she wouldn't take the bottle. When I went back the next day she seemed calm and happy and had taken the bottle over-night. The doctors decided that she was intolerant to something in milk so she's now on the new formula. We then had to switch her from the hospital bottles to a different brand, but luckily she was so hungry she didn't mind. Two weeks on, she's still bottle-feeding happily. I wasn't aiming to transfer her to bottled milk, and it was a sad time for me, but I'm glad the transition was quite smooth.

Teresa from Paddock Wood, mum to Amelie, four, and Juliette, seven months

I've been trying to get my baby to move to bottles for a few weeks now but she's so stubborn – she just doesn't want to know. I end up giving in and feeding her myself. My husband is desperate to feed her himself; I think he feels he's reliant on me always having to take over and it's getting in the way of their bonding. He does do everything else he can – baths, massage and play, but that feed before bed is such a special time and I wish he could get some of that. We've taken a break over the last week as she was getting very worked up and we are hoping to have another go next week. I'm also returning to work soon and really need her on a bottle. I've been enjoying breastfeeding but am now feeling trapped. She's still feeding every three hours, as well as through the night, and I want some sleep!

Sarah from Darlington, mum to Jack, three, and Beth, four months

My daughter fed from both breast and bottle for a couple of months. She had a funny feeding routine that my boobs couldn't handle, taking very little of a morning, but needing a major power feed from 4 p.m. to 8 p.m. I had to start expressing in the mornings as I was leaking so badly. I could then offer her both breasts full when she started her feeding frenzy later in the day, followed by the bottle I'd expressed in the morning. Thankfully, she went for the bottle straight away, no problems. At six months she switched herself exclusively to bottles, mainly all formula by then, when she got a snotty cold, as she obviously found it easier to suck. One good tip if you've been breastfeeding and you want to start offering milk in a bottle is to check the temperature. Breast milk is body temperature, so as similar as possible to that is the best.
Anna from Newton Abbot, mum to Isaac, three, and Milly, two

My son was no problem and would go from boob to bottle and breast milk to formula with no fuss. With my daughter it's been a different story as she would not take a bottle or formula, which meant having to carry on breastfeeding far longer than I really wanted to! I am pro-breastfeeding but think that new mums should be advised to give baby a bottle-feed regularly and fairly early on so they get used to it and then mum can cut down or stop breastfeeding when she is ready to. Health visitors and midwives are often so keen on getting you to breastfeed they forget many women would benefit from being able to share the feeding role.
Michelle from Hitchin, mum to Ed, two, and Evie, eleven months

When my son was born, my plan was to breastfeed for a few weeks then try mixed feeding, but I found that he wouldn't take to a bottle, not even with expressed milk in it. We tried loads of different teats, different baby milks, and even tried feeding him from a spoon. My health visitor wasn't much help as she just kept encouraging me to keep breastfeeding and as a result I carried on until he was eighteen months old. I lost count of the number of times I tried to wean him off my breast and interest him in a bottle. Although I enjoyed the bond of breastfeeding it was draining, as no one could settle him except me. Finally, I went away for a few

days and he stayed with my mum – he had no choice but to drink from a cup then!
Carly from Southend, mum to Dan, three

I have fed both my babies on breastmilk and formula since they were a few weeks old. My son had a very bad tongue tie and didn't feed properly. He had it cut at three weeks by which time my supplies had decreased so I needed the formula to top him up. I fed him at night and morning by breast, and formula for the rest of the time, for four months. My daughter was fine after birth but did feed for hours on end. Unfortunately she didn't gain as much weight as she should and the HV was started to get worried, so I chose to give her a formula top-up too. I'm fortunate that both babies took to the bottle with no problem.
Louisa from Basingstoke, mum to Edward, fifteen months, and Violet, two months

Nothing worked in trying to get our daughter on a bottle, and I was getting desperate as I was due to return to work when she was eight months. I tried just making her wait one day, with help from my dad, but she still wouldn't go for it and after eight hours I had to give in! Finally she took a bottle of expressed milk from my husband and after that she would take one whenever needed, although I carried on breastfeeding too, until she was eighteen months. Another mum I know had a similar problem, but got round it by using a cup and spoon.
Briony from London, mum to Mpilika, three, and Yenga, four months

23 How do I deal with nappy rash?

Nappy rash is common. Your little one is very likely to get it at some point, as it affects up to a third of babies at any given time. It may be mild, and unlikely to cause your baby any real discomfort, or it may be a more severe case, typically characterised by a bright red, livid, spotty rash. It's usually caused when the delicate skin's protective barrier breaks down, allowing the ammonia in urine and bacteria from poo to get into the skin, which is why your baby will be more prone to it when he's ill with diarrhoea. For many babies, there seems to be a connection between nappy rash and teething (see Question 31).

Changing your baby's nappy regularly, and as soon after a poo as possible, and keeping his bottom as clean and dry as you can is the best way to stop nappy rash from flaring up in the first place. It's also a good idea – both by way of prevention and cure – to let your baby spend as much time as is practical without his nappy on, to reduce the amount of time his skin is in contact with wee and poo. Put a large absorbent towel underneath him, try not to worry about the mess, and let him expose his bottom to the world for a while!

What the experts say

Louise says: I'm a big believer in prevention over cure when it comes to nappy rash. So making sure you change your baby's nappy very regularly, and making sure you clean and dry it carefully at each change is vital. I recommend using an inexpensive barrier such as petroleum jelly, or zinc and castor oil ointment, fairly routinely – certainly I'd bung some on at night, when the nappy to skin contact is going to be more prolonged, or at the first signs of any redness or soreness. Nappy-free time whenever possible is a good idea. And getting the right nappy is relevant. Buy the best quality you can afford, so you can be sure it's absorbent, and make sure they fit right – too tight and they could cause chafing, which will worsen nappy rash, too big and they could leak. I know they're convenient, but I usually advise against baby wipes, certainly for very young babies, because even the non-perfumed ones contain ingredients that could be harmful to sensitive bottoms. Cotton wool and water is kinder. You definitely shouldn't use wipes if your baby actually has nappy rash, as they're likely to sting.

When it comes to clearing up nappy rash, there's a wide variety of over-the-counter products, and you should find one is effective. You may find some work better than others and sometimes a product is no help at all. It's a matter of finding out which works best for your baby. If what you suspect is a nappy rash does not clear up quickly, ask your GP to take a look. Sometimes, a fungal or bacterial infection can develop and cause soreness in the area, and may be mistaken for plain old nappy rash. Unfortunately if you treat an infection with nappy rash cream it can make it even worse. Your GP will be able to prescribe a suitable treatment if an infection is the problem.

Occasionally a rash in the area can signal an underlying skin problem such as eczema or allergic dermatitis, triggered by a reaction to a particular substance. If that turns out to be the case, your GP should be able to give you appropriate advice on dealing with it.

What the netmums say

A bit of a bummer

If my two are ever suffering from nappy rash I put talcum powder on the bum after their evening bath, and cover them in Sudocrem. By the morning, they are nearly always better.
Ali from Stratford, mum to Fern and Bailey, nine months

Real nappies and plenty of nappy-free time help prevent nappy rash. If it starts to look red or a bit sore, I just squeeze a bit of breast milk on a clean finger and wipe it on. It definitely promotes healing.
Claire from Southampton, mum to Isobel, seven months

I always put Vaseline on my daughter's bum at most nappy changes, which I think really helps prevent nappy rash. On the few occasions when she has had it, we used Metanium ointment. It's bright yellow and can be messy, but it really did work wonders – any rash would be gone by the morning. If the rash was quite bad I would try to ensure at least an hour of no-nappy time, which can also be rather messy, but definitely seems to help.
Carrie from Manchester, mum to Ellyna, twenty-two months

To prevent nappy rash in the first place, I recommend very regular nappy changes and fragrance-free wipes.
Julie from Lichfield, mum to Eve, twelve, Charlie, two, and Amy, seven months

Cotton wool and water, plain water baths, and a product called Simmons Pawpaw Salve have always worked for us. Pawpaw Salve is a natural, fruit-based ointment that is really popular in Australia and New Zealand but is still fairly unknown in the UK, so I've only ever been able to order it online. I find zinc-based creams seem to make the problem worse.
Mandy from Wakefield, mum to Daniel, six months

I never experienced nappy rash with my first, but my second little boy has sensitive skin and whenever he got an upset tummy, all the dirty nappies caused his little bum to become red and angry-looking. A friend discovered a product called Cheeky Wipes online, and recommended them. They're reusable wipes, soaked in chamomile and lavender. At first I was sceptical but they cleared up the rash within a day or two and I was totally won over.
Jo from Glasgow, mum to Seth, six, and Jude, eleven months

Lots of fresh air is the best thing for nappy rash. Easier said than done, I know, but it really helps, both in terms of prevention and cure. I usually leave my little one's nappy off after a poo, at least then you'll only have to clean up pee at worst. Also make sure your baby's bottom is completely dry, for instance if you've been using wet wipes, before you put a nappy back on.
Karen from Glasgow, mum to Cameron, two

When my little one has nappy rash, I always followed my mum's recommendation – put a spoonful of bicarbonate of soda in a bath or basin of warm water, and dip your baby's bottom in it. It's really good for soothing angry skin.
Maggie from Reigate, mum to Catherine, two

I asked my pharmacist about my son's severe nappy rash, which looked red and 'scabby', and he recommended a thin layer of Canesten anti-fungal cream. It cleared up so much faster than it ever had before with a regular nappy rash cream.
Phillipa from Swindon, mum to Toby, fourteen months

My little girl recently had terrible nappy rash due to diarrhoea from a tummy bug. Her bottom was blistered and red raw. I took her to the doctors, who suggested air-time and Sudocrem, but it didn't help. Then a friend gave this advice and it cleared up within two days: wash with warm water – just your hands, no cotton wool – so either dunk baby in the basin, or if old enough, get them to stand up in the shower. Then dab dry with a towel, lie them on the bed and use the hairdryer on a very low heat on the skin for a couple of minutes until completely dry. After a few minutes nappy-free time, apply Metanium ointment. Worked a treat!
Louise from Stevenage, mum to Hannah, twenty months

Happily, my son has never had nappy rash. I don't use any wipes on his bum at all, just cotton wool and a bit of lotion, and I honestly believe that's why. His bum is always smooth, smells good and just does not get sore. I think it's because the lotion absorbs into the skin as opposed to being damp from wipes.

Vanessa from Peterborough, mum to Laila, five, and Nathan, six months

24 What should I do about constipation?

A baby suffering from constipation can cause a lot of worry: after all, it's a painful business. Constipation causes the stools (poo) to be hard, making it difficult for a baby to pass a motion. You'll probably be able to tell she's constipated by the look on her face and the extreme effort she seems to be making when trying to 'go'.

Don't assume your baby is constipated simply because she hasn't had a poo for a long time, as it's very variable how often individual babies may go. Better indications of constipation to watch for are obvious 'straining', a solid abdomen, and the appearance of hard or pellet-like stools when she *does* manage to go. It's a good idea to consult your health visitor, or better still, go straight to your GP, who may want to prescribe treatment that will stop your baby suffering – and before the problem is compounded, and becomes worse.

What the experts say

Louise says: It's not unheard of, but in my experience constipation is unusual in breastfed babies, because breast milk is so easily digested, and the stools are softer. What can often happen is that parents think their baby is suffering from constipation because she hasn't had a poo for several days or more. But actually, it's not abnormal for a baby to go that long without a poo and in itself, the absence of a bowel movement doesn't necessarily mean a baby is constipated. A constipated baby's poo will be hard and pellet-like, and that's how you know the difference. She may also become rather distressed when trying to go for a poo and may even end up with a little tear, or anal fissure, which may be painful for her but can soothed with a little medicated cream.

For relief of constipation, I would recommend offering your baby an ounce of cooled, boiled water in a bottle or a sippy cup, in between her normal milk feeds. I personally wouldn't advise giving fruit juice or sugar water to babies below weaning age – water alone should do the job as well, and you risk giving her a taste for sweet things. Gently massaging her abdomen can also be effective in getting the digestive system moving. Use a clock-wise motion, which means you'll be working in the direction of the intestine. You could also try moving your baby's legs in a 'cycling' motion.

Make sure you're making up formula feeds as directed, as too much powder can be a cause of constipation. And do be wary of using 'hungry baby' or stage two brands before your baby is ready. Generally speaking, it may be worth switching formulas to see if that helps – some babies object when you do this, others don't mind at all. In any case, it could be worth a try.

During and after weaning, both formula-fed and breastfed babies may experience constipation, as their digestive systems adjust to the new composition of their food. Offering extra fruit purée or fruit juice, one part diluted with ten parts water, can help get things moving. Prune juice is particularly good. And offering extra water to drink remains good advice – although it's important only to offer water as a supplement to, not a replacement for, regular milk feeds, which babies continue to need up to the age of one. I'd still steer clear of sugar water as a constipation cure, though, as it just seems unnecessary.

You can get laxative medication over the counter, but I would always recommend consulting your doctor first before trying these. It is a good idea, though, to jump on constipation problems quite quickly once they arise – and if the recommendations outlined above aren't getting you anywhere after a day or two, I would see your GP, who may want to prescribe treatment. If constipation is left, your baby's likely to become uncomfortable, windy and grizzly, and – a bit further down the line still – it may start to affect her appetite, or cause vomiting.

Dr David says: In most cases, constipation in babies is what's known as 'idiopathic'. It means there's no particular cause, and it's just one of those things. But once a baby becomes constipated and it hurts to try and have a poo, she may try and hold on to it, and the result is a vicious circle because it hardens and then becomes even more difficult for her to pass. Potential symptoms you might see in your baby include straining or obvious pain when doing a poo, anal tears (fissures) and bleeding, or poo that resembles rabbit droppings.

In the first instance, it's worth asking your health visitor for advice about how you can help your constipated baby at home, but in general I'd advise talking to your GP sooner rather than later – early treatment with laxatives is often advisable, to ensure the problem doesn't deteriorate. If your baby's suffered from constipation from birth or during the first few weeks of life, or if alongside any constipation she's not gaining weight or is vomiting and has a bloated tummy, or if the treatment you have been prescribed for constipation isn't helping after three months, you should ask for a referral to a specialist.

What the netmums say

Trouble going

My daughter had problems pooing since birth. Sometimes she would go without one for over a week! The problem became worse when she was prescribed medicine for her reflux. We were then given a laxative solution to help her, but decided that what was best was to stop all medications and let her return to her natural routine and deal with the reflux symptoms rather than her being so bunged up. The whole problem eased when we started weaning, and my daughter went from being an erratic, once-every-three-days pooer to having one once a day or every other day.
Caroline from Manchester, mum to Natalia, ten months

Riley suffered with constipation from around three months, on and off. By five months he was only going every other day and it was obviously painful, so our health visitor suggested weaning him a little early to see if some veg would help. We tried everything, from massage to prune juice, grapes and a vegetarian diet, but nothing helped, and it just got worse. By six months he was screaming and shaking every time he went – it was heartbreaking! The doctor prescribed a laxative solution, Lactulose, but there was no improve-ment. We were told to 'give it a month', and that he would 'grow out of it', but still there was no improvement. Eventually, when he was nine months, we went to see a different doctor, whose own daughter had also suffered with constipation. She put him on a stronger laxative medication – it instantly worked and we were so relieved!
Hannah from Stratford-upon-Avon, mum to Riley, two

My daughter became constipated at six weeks. We were advised not to change her milk but to try extra water, or water with some orange juice in it. She refused both but was in agony and even ended up with an anal fissure. She would strain so much she was sick, and her poos were like concrete pebbles. We changed to a different formula milk, Aptamil Comfort, and within forty-eight hours she was sorted.
Natasha from Redditch, mum to Annabelle, four months

Unfortunately, my wee boy had a phase of being quite constipated. He'd go days without a dirty nappy and when he did it was really hard and painful for him. He ended up with little fissures, which was awful. I was exclusively breastfeeding, so it was really stressing me out because you read that booby babies are not likely to become constipated. We treated him with stomach massages and put a little bit of Vaseline on his bottom to prevent the fissures. Ultimately, the 'cure' seemed to be when I gave up dairy. He has a milk protein allergy, and the dairy passing through my breast milk must have been irritating his stomach. If your baby's showing signs of constipation, I advise taking him into a warm bath with you, and tummy rubbing in there. If there's an accident, it's easy enough to disinfect the bath.
Marianne from Uddingston, mum to William, twenty-two months

My daughter has terrible constipation – she screams and screams when she's trying to pass a stool. It's miserable for me, and for her. She has medication from the doctor, but she needs it every single day. It doesn't seem like a great idea to me, but every time we try to cut it back she gets stopped up again. Before she had the medication, she would go for two or three days without pooping, then there'd be some runny poop throughout the day, and finally she would clear out, with much screaming. The last couple of days of the cycle she would hardly eat. We know when she's getting backed up because of the not eating.
Susannah from York, mum to Eleanor, fourteen months

When my second daughter had bad constipation that lasted for a few weeks, I found that putting her on her back and 'pumping' her legs was the only thing that worked for her. I also tried changing her formula, and it eventually stopped, thank goodness. But their poor little faces when they can't go. It's terrible.
Siobhan from Walton, mum to Lucy, five, and Kim, two

My little one is exclusively breastfed but even so, as a newborn he suffered really severe constipation, going without a poo for over four weeks. All the health professionals kept telling me it was OK and it would sort itself out, but it didn't. At his six-week check, the doctor referred us to hospital immediately, having explained that there are a few rare but serious conditions that are linked to constipation. He was examined, X-rayed, scanned and had blood tests taken, which was all really scary, although the staff were great and Edward was very brave. Thankfully, the results ruled out any serious conditions, as well as allergies or intolerances to anything I was eating. But they couldn't really give an explanation. For now, all they can do is prescribe laxatives and occasional suppositories to manage the symptoms. Calpol also helps ease the pain. However, the basic problem remains unsolved.
Clare from Portsmouth, mum to Edward, three months

Niamh was constipated during the second week of her life. She really struggled to pass a stool and when she did it was a hard, dry pellet. I got concerned about her when she lost interest in drinking her milk. She was admitted to hospital overnight and given an enema, which worked. After that, my health visitor recommended changing her formula milk to SMA because it contains some enzymes that help with digestion, and after that we didn't have so many problems with constipation. My first daughter has Down's Syndrome and children with this condition tend to suffer a little more from constipation. She had problems when I started weaning her but as she hated water I ended up giving her very diluted fruit juice, just to ensure that she was properly hydrated. And I found that tinned prunes in her cereal every morning worked wonders.

Lucy from Neston, mum to Ciara, five, and Greg and Niamh, three

We had a nightmare with our third daughter, who was constipated big time from three weeks old. She'd go red and scream the house down when trying to poop, and had bad tummy pains that made the crying worse. I took her to the doctors and they said the usual: give her water between feeds and once she was old enough, a spoonful of orange juice or prune juice. No luck! At about eight months we were given lactulose solution, but with still no success – she was going once every four to five days. Her poo was rock solid and her little bum would bleed. Doctors then prescribed a medication called Movicol. This took a few sachets to work and basically gave her diarrhoea, but at least she was cleared out. It worked for a couple of months, but it was a nightmare to get it down her. Then we were prescribed suppositories. They were horrible for her, but it worked. We found that once she was potty-trained, at three, the constipation went. I guess she was mature enough to understand the more she held it in, the more it would hurt.

Aimee from Chester, mum to Lauren and Megan, six, and Sophie, five

25 What are all those funny noises?

At first, the only noise you're likely to get from your baby is crying. But before long you should start to hear all sorts of lovely sounds in the form of coos and gurgles. This is the start of your baby's talking skills developing, and a way for him to practise the movements of the lips, palate and tongue that he'll need to form proper speech later on. He'll then discover consonant sounds like 'b' and 'd', and somewhere between four and nine months, typically, he'll start to join vowel and consonant sounds together repetitively – it's known as 'babbling', and you're likely to hear a lot of it as he experiments with the sounds he can make. After a while, he'll start to babble with tone and rhythm, so that it sounds for all the world like he's conversing in sentences.

Among your baby's early babbles, you may well make out the sounds 'da-da' and 'ma-ma'. It's a particularly lovely noise for parents to hear – but the truth is, these are simply two of the most common consonant sounds, and among the easiest for him to copy. He won't start to use them with real meaning for a while yet (for more on talking, see Question 44) but meanwhile, your delighted response will help him make the connection. Don't forget to stop and listen, and to talk back when your baby 'talks' to you. Experts say it's the most important thing you can do to boost his communication skills.

What the experts say

Maggie says: It's a happy milestone when your baby starts communicating with all those lovely coos and gurgles, and then, a bit later, the tuneful babbling. After all, it's the beginnings of his speech and language development. Listening to your baby and joining in the 'conversation' by copying his noises is a great way to bond with him, and a vital way to boost his language and social skills. Making eye contact and showing him lots of different facial expressions is important too. It's because of this that many experts are concerned about forward-facing push-chairs, which make it very difficult to respond to and communicate with your baby while out and about – if your baby has one of these, try to find plenty of other opportunities in the day to chat with him. And if he has a dummy, I'd advise keeping it tucked away as much as possible during the day, as speech therapists are concerned that over-use can interfere with babbling and other language-development skills.

As with all the milestones, different babies will begin babbling at different stages. I'd be inclined to mention it to a health professional if a baby was not babbling by nine months. And if your baby stops babbling, having babbled earlier on, it's defi-nitely worth consulting a GP, as it could indicate a hearing problem.

What the netmums say

Say that again

Kobey makes lots of very cute noises and even seems to have proper 'chats' with his toys! It started with a lot of 'aaahs' and then there were a lot of what seemed to be 'yehs', and a couple of 'da-das' – but to date, no 'ma-mas', much to my husband's joy! I sit and chat to him at all opportunities, and always take his 'babbling' as an indication that he's joining in!
Janine from Caerphilly, mum to Kobey, eight months

My daughter coos and makes 'ba-ba-ba' noises, but by far her favourite noise is screaming – not a crying scream, but a high-pitched 'I'm so happy and excited' kind of scream! It's funny, but very odd. When we're at playgroup, other adults seem shocked and want to know how I put up with it, but honestly, it's totally

different to a tired or upset scream. My friend's son cries whenever she does it, purely because it's so loud!
Caroline from Manchester, mum to Natalia, ten months

Harry has just started to really coo. You can have a great conversation with him! Just a minute ago I was talking to him about what I can ask his daddy for, and it sounded like he said 'car'! Of course, I know he didn't, but it was so funny.
Rachel from Skipton, mum to Harry, two months

My son began cooing at about four and a half months, making 'aaaahm', 'maaa', and 'ooooeeeeeh' sounds, then started alternating his tone a lot more so it sounds like he's conversing with you. He then discovered a high-pitched scream, which he made whenever he was happy! And today he's started something different, just repeating the same low tone sounds a few times before squealing. I spend as much time as I can sitting with him, playing and talking. My mum told me the other day I started talking early and I'm really hoping he will be the same. I won't be disappointed if he doesn't but I am so looking forward to having real conversations with him.
Pam from Arklow, mum to Ruairí, seven months

My twin girls are hilarious! They sit babbling away to each other, mainly shouting 'ah, ah, ah', or 'dadadadadadadada'. They do say 'ma-ma' a lot too, and have done for a few months. They both also say 'Ganda', which is our dog – Gandalf. I'm convinced they're talking to each other, because they have big grins and giggles while they do it. I always join in their conversations. It adds to the hilarity.
Cat from Edinburgh, mum to George, six, and Freyja and Tavia, eleven months

Oliver's been a 'talker' from day one. He chattered away to his toys on the change table and loved to get up close and personal with his teddies. Now he still chatters and babbles away to himself, and anyone who is listening. He even raises his voice when making a point and has the most amazing facial expressions to go with it! He particularly loves sitting on his granddad's knee and will chatter

on for ages as though he's relaying everything that's happened in his day. He has a wonderful repertoire of sounds, from squeals to chortles to 'rahhhhs'. I can't wait until he is talking properly just to know what he is saying.
Kylie from Bedford, mum to Jared, thirteen, and Oliver, nineteen months

Harriet seems to have always made noises either in annoyance or happiness. She does plenty of chatting, mostly making 'da-da-da dow-dow' noises and she has a sound that she uses specially for her sisters which is more of a vowel sound, but don't ask me to write it! She also sings beautifully and very tunefully, but she has no actual words yet, although she'll make a good attempt to copy you if you say a word for her. She also 'reads' with enthusiasm, turning pages and babbling as she does so!
Juliette from Harrogate, mum to Emily-Anne, six, Olivia, four, and Harriet, eleven months

It was lovely when my son started cooing at two and a half months. I made a recording of it and now it's my ring tone! I talked, and still talk, to him a lot. His started to say 'da-da-da-da' and 'na-na-na-na' at seven months. And when I sing to him, he certainly lets us hear his vocals.
Sylvia from Watford, mum to Zachary, eight months

My little one has been babbling away for the past two or three months. He says 'da-da' quite a lot and he chats away to his sister, and screams and laughs lots. I've spoken to all my babies from birth and I'm sure that's why my older two were talking in full sentences by eighteen months. It's still hard now to get a word in (but I wouldn't have it any other way).
Tracey from Burnley, mum to Daniel, eighteen, Olivia, ten, and Harrison, seven months

26 What should I do if she's poorly?

It's a miserable situation when your baby is unwell. Unfortunately, babies have underdeveloped immune systems that make them vulnerable to minor illness, so it's a situation you can probably expect to find yourself in more than once when she's small. Often, you'll be able to look after your poorly baby at home, with some extra care and attention. But it may not always be obvious when you can do that and when you should get her checked out.

Always seek help if you're worried. Any decent GP should be happy to take a look at your baby just to be on the safe side, or at least to chat to you on the phone about it. It's also worth knowing what your other options are in terms of health services in your area. Is it an issue that your health visitor could advise on? Could your surgery's nurse practitioner help? You may also have a walk-in centre or drop-in clinic in your area – if you haven't already worked out where it is, and when it's open, now's the time to do so. And don't forget NHS Direct (NHS 24 in Scotland), which you can telephone for advice, twenty-four hours a day. It goes without saying that in an emergency, or if you're deeply concerned about your baby's health, and you can't get hold of a doctor, you should take her to the nearest A&E department, or dial 999 and ask for an ambulance.

What the experts say

Louise says: When you become a mum for the first time it's natural to be filled with anxiety, particularly if your baby's health is below par. It's a normal parental response. You might find yourself wondering if you really need to take her to the doctor or not – some mums even worry that they'll be seen as 'neurotic' if they seek medical help too frequently, or for no good reason. My advice, generally speaking, is that if you think there's something wrong with your baby's health, get her seen. Sometimes it will be based on a gut feeling that something isn't quite right – perhaps her cry is different, she's not interested in feeding, isn't as responsive as usual, or just isn't herself. Your instinct as a parent will generally be right. Most health services have a good understanding of that and hopefully you would never be turned away if you were worried, particularly if your baby is very young. She should have priority at most surgeries – if not, you may have to be a bit assertive. In any case, you don't ever have to feel guilty, or that you're being neurotic, if you need to get your baby checked out! Health professionals are paid to provide a service; they're not doing it from the kindness of their hearts. If you're regularly having trouble getting a speedy appointment for your baby, then maybe you need to think about changing your GP. At the very least, you should be able to get a telephone consultation, and sometimes, that's all you need to put your mind at rest. NHS Direct is also a great service for worried parents, especially out of hours. They'll take you through a flow chart of symptoms and should either be able to reassure you, or advise you to see a doctor when possible. And if they think the situation sounds urgent, they'll pass you on to the ambulance service.

Some minor illnesses, like colds, can of course be treated at home with a bit of extra care. It's thought that most babies will come down with ten colds, on average, during their first year, which is actually a good thing, because it helps to build up their immunity. There's not a lot you can do about them, other than offering extra feeds and perhaps extra water to drink. If she can't feed because of a blocked nose, it's worth seeing your GP, or asking your pharmacist about saline drops which can help unblock it.

Fever control is also important with babies as high temperatures can result in what's called a febrile convulsion, or fit. In children under the age of five, a fever is a temperature that's over 37.2°C if measured under the armpit, 37.8°C orally or 38°C if measured in the ear, on the forehead or rectally. Babies over three months can be given the appropriate dose of an infant antipyretic (fever-reducing) medicine, such as paracetamol or ibuprofen. You can also help by keeping her cool, perhaps removing a layer or two of clothes and cooling her with a wet sponge – use tepid, rather than cold water. Although a fever is a common symptom of many mild illnesses and can usually be treated at home, it can also signal more serious conditions, so it's important to keep a close eye on a baby with a high temperature and to be alert to any other symptoms she has at the same time. Where a baby under three months is concerned, I would always suggest seeking medical advice on a fever, regardless.

Tummy bugs that cause vomiting or diarrhoea, or both, will usually come and go within a day or two. Although there's not too much to be done about them at the time, they can cause dehydration, so your doctor may prescribe a rehydration solution to replace lost fluids. If vomiting is projectile, bloody, green or bile-like, consult your GP, and equally, if diarrhoea is blood-streaked, that's something you should get checked out.

Rashes can make parents panic. Usually they'll be harmless, often appearing after recovery from a virus, but a spreading, blotchy purple rash that doesn't fade under pressure is a potential sign of meningococcal septicaemia (blood poisoning caused by the same type of bacteria that can cause meningitis) and needs medical attention immediately. Rolling a glass over a rash is a simple but effective test – if the rash *doesn't* lose colour or fade, get help straight away. Of course, if a rash appears and it's worrying you, you may want to get it checked out at the first opportunity anyway, for peace of mind.

It's rare for a baby to be dangerously ill, thankfully, but some symptoms should put you on 'red alert'. If she's not breathing or having problems breathing, has had a convulsion (a fit) when she has never had one before, seems floppy, limp or unresponsive, or is unconscious or semi-conscious, will not wake, or appears not to recognise you, dial 999 or get her promptly to the nearest A&E department.

What the netmums say

Doctor, doctor

I tend to take them in when I feel that there's something a GP can actually do to help. A slight sniffle, a cough or a fever simply isn't treatable by a doctor. They can only offer Calpol, which we already have in the cupboard. However if an infection has set in, or the fever is out of control, or they're obviously becoming dehydrated, well then, I know my little ones need help. I think that often, GPs don't mean to be impatient with mums; it's just their frustration at only being able to offer limited help for most colds and flu.
Taliah from Worcester, mum to Kaydence, six, Aurelia, four, Nymeria, two, and Octavian, ten months

My daughter has no hope, as I'm a primary school teacher and bring home all sorts of germs. I always seek help when she is ill. Generally I would use the NHS Direct website or call them first. I've had to take her to the doctor's three times and had bad service on each occasion. The first time was after she had an abnormal reaction to her TB injection [which is offered to babies in some high-risk areas] – the advisor on NHS Direct kept telling me it was normal, but I stuck with my instincts and got an out-of-hours appointment late that evening, which it turned out I was right to do. The second and third times have been over conjunctivitis. Trying to get an appointment on the same day at my GP surgery is like trying to find gold in your back garden – even when I've stressed it's for a baby. My doctor told me that as a first-time parent I worried too much, but that I should have brought her in sooner about the conjunctivitis. You can't win!
Louise from Luton, mum to Caitlyn, ten months

We had a fright with our son when he came out in a purple rash. My husband checked it with a glass and it didn't go away, so we phoned NHS 24 and they told us to go straight to hospital and keep him awake. We were met by a doctor at the door who checked him over and admitted him straight away. Thankfully it turned out to be nothing serious, just the result of a virus. I recently

used NHS 24 again and found that they responded very quickly and put me straight through to a doctor. I couldn't praise the response we received enough. All in all, I've been reassured and impressed by our healthcare services. I have always been told that a doctor would rather offer reassurance than have an illness go unchecked. I would go with self-care as far as possible, but would always seek advice if I was worried.
Miriam from Aberdeen, mum to Charlie, fourteen months

If ever I'm worried, I get on the phone to NHS Direct. My oldest son was once very hot, very sleepy and sort of lifeless, and when I phoned NHS Direct, they sent an ambulance round for me. In hospital he was monitored for a bit, and given medicine. There was nothing badly wrong with him as it turned out, it was a perfectly common illness, but as he was my first, I was very glad to take the professionals' advice.
Kate from Shrewsbury, mum to Jack, eight, and Charlie, two

Instinct usually guides me, but if I'm unsure I will ask my mum's advice, and also use an online forum which is an absolute godsend if you have a worry that you feel stupid asking a health professional about. In my experience as a first-time mum, I sometimes get the vibe from the GPs that I am worrying about nothing. However, I hardly ever take her to the doctor's, so it's not as though I take her at the slightest snuffle!
Amanda from Fleet, mum to Tabitha, nine months

At eleven days old, my son developed a high temperature and started projectile vomiting his feeds. At first I was concerned, but everyone kept telling me it was probably just a bad belly. I left it for a few hours and then he brought up his next feed in the same way, and I just knew it wasn't right. When I rang my midwife, she also said it was probably just a bad belly and actually told me I was being paranoid! I rang my out-of-hours service and they said they would check him over to reassure me. They then told me to take him straight to the children's hospital. It turns out he had developed a urinary tract infection and septicaemia, either of which could have killed him at his age. He was in hospital for five days and had numerous tests afterwards to make sure it wasn't caused by an underlying problem. As a mum, I think you *know* when something isn't right with your baby and sometimes you have to make a real nuisance of yourself to get your child (especially your first child) seen by professionals.

Jessica from Bristol, mum to Marley, two

I usually use my instinct, or ask my mum's advice. But if I feel something's not right I would not hesitate to see my GP. If they say nothing's wrong, then great, but if something *is* wrong I'll have done the right thing. I was always told, if in doubt get your child checked and don't ever feel you're wasting the doctor's time. They are there to help.

Amanda from Doncaster, mum to Maddie, two

Generally in the first instance I would check the symptoms with my online friends, to see if anyone else has experienced the same symptoms and what they did. I'd ring NHS Direct if it seemed mild but, if in doubt, would see the doctor.

Emma from Banbury, mum to Nathaniel, four months

27 Is it safe for him to be immunised?

Your baby will be invited to have the first in a series of routine immunisations at two months, followed by further sessions at three and four months. Along with a set of 'booster' jabs at twelve or thirteen months (plus a set later, just before starting school), these injections will offer him protection against a number of highly dangerous diseases: diphtheria, tetanus, whooping cough (pertussis), polio, Haemophilus influenzae type b (Hib), pneumococcal infection, and meningitis C. Your baby will also be offered immunisation against measles, mumps and rubella, better known as the MMR. Health professionals will urge you to take up all these injections, at the times recommended. They are in no doubt that all the immunisations currently offered are safe and effective – and that it's important for your baby to be immunised as early as possible, as it's the very young that are most at risk of being seriously harmed by these diseases. And it's not just about your own baby's health: immunisation protects the wider community, too.

Not all parents are comfortable with the idea of vaccinations. Some fear that too many vaccines could 'overload' a young baby's system; others worry specifically about possible adverse reactions. In particular, a major scare over the MMR vaccine that suggested a link to the development of autism some years ago – despite being discredited since – has left lingering worries for some. It's not at all unreasonable to feel anxious, and to want your questions about vaccinations answered. Do give it some time, thought and research, if that's what you need to feel reassured. No one can ever promise you that immunisation is 100 per cent risk-free, but the evidence is overwhelmingly in its favour as the safer option for your child.

What the experts say

Louise says: You should automatically be offered an appointment for your baby's first lot of jabs at the time they're due – however, you may not necessarily get a reminder about subsequent injections due, so it's a good idea to know what the schedule involves and when. Don't forget to take your 'red book' when you go, so the jabs can be recorded in it. If someone else takes your baby, you'll need to send in your written consent.

Choose clothes that can easily be removed or rolled-up for the appointment. And try not to feel stressed – they're simple to perform and any discomfort is fleeting. Some babies barely even notice what's going on. For the majority, there will be no adverse reaction following vaccination, but sometimes the injected area can become sore or swollen, or a baby will develop a mild fever, which you'll probably be advised to treat with an appropriate dose of infant paracetamol or ibuprofen, and by keeping him cool. He may be irritable and miserable for a day or two. Very rarely indeed, a high temperature can lead to a febrile convulsion, or fit, which is why you'll probably be asked to sit in the waiting room for a few minutes afterwards, just as a precaution. You'll be advised to postpone your child's jab if he is ill and has a fever – but there's no need to avoid them in the case of a minor illness if there's no fever present. There's also no reason to avoid any of the routine vaccinations in the UK programme if your child has asthma, eczema or allergies. Don't worry if you miss an appointment – it doesn't mean you'll have to start a course all over again. Just make another as soon as possible.

If your baby was born pre-term, bear in mind that it's even more important he gets his vaccinations on time, as premmies are at greater risk from infection and also have immune systems that are less developed. In fact, some pre-term babies receive their first set of immunisations whilst still in the special care unit.

I didn't hesitate to get my own daughter vaccinated against everything possible, and I'm always confident in urging parents to go ahead with immunisation because I know the schedule we have is based on good scientific evidence. These jabs are offered to protect your child – and others in the wider community – from getting potentially life-threatening diseases. If you're nervous and you want more information, ask your health visitor, who should be happy to point you in the direction of more detailed facts.

Dr David says: As a consultant paediatrician, I am very much pro-immunisation, and absolutely convinced it's the right thing for parents to take up all the routine jabs that are offered. As with all medicines, vaccines have to be thoroughly tested before they can be licensed and used, and even then their use will continue to be closely monitored, more so than any drug. And as with all medicines, vaccines can have side effects. But serious problems that are proven to be directly linked to them are extremely rare indeed. Any risk is massively outweighed by the health benefits of being protected by immunisation against a range of illnesses that can have devastating consequences for health, including brain damage, disabilities and deadly infections and, in some cases, can kill.

You shouldn't fear that your baby could be 'overloaded' by vaccines. A child's immune system naturally protects against thousands of different germs and can cope easily with multiple vaccines at this age. And as far as the MMR vaccine is concerned, there really is no evidence to support a link between it and autism. Worldwide consensus is that it's safe, and in fact, the National Autism Society ensures parents get their child immunised against MMR. Some parents want to know if paying to have the MMR administered in three single vaccines – since the NHS don't offer this – rather than all at once is a safer option, but there's no evidence that it's safer and in fact, the delay between each vaccine just leaves children unprotected for longer. We know the MMR is effective, as it's been studied so thoroughly all around the world, whereas the use of single vaccines hasn't. It's also a myth – and a dangerous one – that homeopathy or other 'natural' alternatives can offer your baby the same protection that immunisation can. The fact is, there's no other option to protect your child from these diseases if you do not immunise, apart from luck.

And that luck is dependent on most other parents getting their babies vaccinated – so if you hope others do, why shouldn't you?

Rarely, vaccines can result in mild, local reactions such as acute swelling or a red itchy rash. You should speak to your GP if this occurs, but it doesn't necessarily rule out further doses. Even more rarely – about once in every million cases – a severe or 'anaphylactic' reaction is caused, and GP surgeries have the equipment to deal with this rare eventuality. Vaccines often result in your child having a temperature but that's a normal response, since they work by fooling the baby's immune system into thinking they have the infection, so that antibodies will be created that will automatically offer protection against that infection in the future. Even if your baby seems poorly afterwards, the effect will never be as great as actually having the infection because the bug's been introduced in a weaker form – which is why children need to be given most vaccines several times, to ensure long-term protection.

I'd always advise any parent considering not immunising their child to think hard, to look into it carefully, and to speak to other people. If you have questions about vaccinations, that's entirely reasonable, and it's important you take time to have them properly answered before making that decision. But be aware that there's a lot of conflicting information out there, particularly online, and not all of it is based on concrete scientific evidence – which the case *for* immunisation is.

What the netmums say

Protective measures

I knew vaccination was the right thing to do. The most both my children have done is cry a little afterwards. It's not really that big a deal. The worst one was the pre-school booster as my son was more aware of what was happening, but he got over it.
Teresa from Long Eaton, mum to Daniel, five, and Ruth, eleven months

My little one has had all the immunisations available on the NHS. I'm still hearing of people not allowing their kids to have the MMR jab, because of the research linking it with autism, despite it being proven false. I heard a father on the news ages ago claiming that his son must have 'caught' autism from the MMR, because his other son hasn't had the MMR and doesn't have autism. People should look into these things before putting their child at risk.

Amy from Croydon, mum to Penny, twenty-one months

I've found this the hardest issue as a mother. I'm from a family where many of us have not been vaccinated, or had a select few vaccines, and although between us we have experienced rubella, whooping cough and measles, none of these things proved to be serious. I will have a much stronger immunity now, and one that is natural. So I believe some vaccines are not necessary for all. My daughter has just had tetanus and diphtheria and will have polio next year, as I do have concerns over these, even though they are extremely rare. But I was not prepared to give my daughter all the jabs, particularly all in one go, at such a young age. I do not take this issue lightly though, and have spent a long time researching it. It bothers me that the number of vaccinations has increased so much over the last few decades, and that they are having so many together, and so young. I do feel a good diet and lifestyle has a big impact. It may not stop some unfortunate illness, but will certainly give you a much better immunity.

Katie from Leek, mum to Mia, nineteen months

All four of my children have been, or are currently being, immunised. I do not worry at all about the 'chemicals' in the vaccines, because it is a small sacrifice to make – and over a lifetime we process billions of chemicals. And the brief moment of suffering at the clinic, when they get the jab, is nothing compared to the diseases themselves and their possible side effects. Immunising my children also helps protect others with low or no immunity, such as transplant patients, those undergoing chemotherapy, newborn babies and elderly people.

Willow from Loughborough, mum to Sacha, eleven, Tabitha, four, Theo, two, and Barney, four months

My daughter has had all her jabs. I weighed up the pros and cons and decided it was best. So far, no damage done. I understand there are small risks with immunisations, but isn't that the same with any medication? Jabs aren't pleasant but as long as they protect against these diseases then my daughter and any future children will have them. But it's a personal choice. I would not judge those who choose not to immunise.

Katie from Nantwich, mum to Isabelle, eighteen months

I used to blame MMR for my eldest son's autism as his behaviour became problematic around that time – and what with the media circus that surrounded [the now-discredited research], I did start to wonder. Looking back, though, he's *always* been autistic, it's just that it wasn't a 'problem' until he started being of an age where he was expected to fit in and socialise. Before that he was a little angel, albeit in his own little world.

Alison from Wellingborough, mum to Kyle, nine, Dexter, three, and Lucas, sixteen months

I hated taking my babies for their jabs. It's so against what you feel as a mother to hold your tiny baby still while someone stabs her with a needle. I read up on it, to make sure I was making an evidence-based decision each time, but I couldn't find an argument against vaccinating that was as compelling as the one for public health. My nagging sense of social responsibility trumped everything else. How would I feel if my kids got away with a mild dose of measles, but the poor kid they inadvertently passed it on to ended up with a more serious case? Bloody awful, that's how. I have two robust kids who barely reacted to any of their jabs and, while I usually try to keep them away from unnecessary substances like additives or pesticides, when it came to jabs, I gritted my teeth and went ahead.

Hilary from Sheffield, mum to Isobel, five, and Caitlin, two

Neither of my two children have had the MMR yet. They have had single vaccines, although my daughter has gone without the single mumps vaccine, as it's not available in the UK any more. I have three autoimmune diseases, all of which developed after my own vaccinations, as a child. I've done a lot of careful research into the subject, and found studies that show where the mother has, in particular, autoimmune thyroid disease, there is increased risk of adverse reaction from the MMR, and early onset autoimmune disease in the child. I showed my GP the research, and he agreed that in my situation he would have gone for single jabs, too. I get angry when people say that mums who opt for single vaccines are stupid.

Sheridan from Chatteris, mum to Seth, four, and Stella, three

I see vaccinations the same way I see brushing children's teeth, or disciplining them when they do something dangerous. These are all things that aren't pleasant to do, but they prevent things that are even more unpleasant happening in the future.

Abi from Mitcham, mum to Alice, eight, Byron, five, and Phoenix, eight months

I'm completely in favour of vaccinations. I didn't give the MMR vaccine a second thought and always knew that Freya was having it, along with all the others. I had them, and it didn't do me any harm. However, I do feel that the issue can be confusing for parents – especially new mums – because there's conflicting information out there, making it hard to make an informed decision.

Anita from Swindon, mum to Freya, eighteen months

28 How can I prevent 'flat head syndrome'?

If your baby seems to be developing a flat back, or side, to her head, it's nothing to panic about. It's likely to be caused by a painless disorder known as positional plagiocephaly – also known sometimes as 'flat head syndrome'. It happens because a baby's skull – which is made up of plates of bone that are not joined at first, but gradually fuse together as she grows – is still soft and can be misshapen by pressure. This may happen in the womb, but often it happens when a baby lies or sits very frequently in one position.

Positional plagiocephaly is common these days, affecting as many as half of babies to some degree or other. The rise in cases is undoubtedly because babies these days are put to sleep on their backs – quite rightly, as it's a significant factor in reducing the risk of Sudden Infant Death or cot death – and perhaps too because of the amount of time they tend to spend in car seats and bouncers. Babies born pre-term are particularly prone to it because their skulls are even softer. In most cases, flattened heads will gradually revert to a more normal shape during a baby's first year and beyond, and there are simple repositioning techniques you can take to boost this improvement. Some parents seek more intensive treatment in the form of a remoulding helmet or head band. These aren't available on the NHS, so if it's something you're considering, you'll need to be prepared to pay. It's also advisable to get one fitted sooner rather than later, ideally before six or seven months.

What the experts say

Louise says: Prevention is better than cure when it comes to positional plagiocephaly, so it's a good idea, from the start, to employ some simple measures to protect against flat head syndrome. It's also a good idea to take action as soon as you notice any sort of flattening, before it has a chance to get any worse.

Try to let your baby have as much 'tummy time' as possible during the day, and to keep stretches in bouncy chairs and car seats to a minimum. If your baby tends to rest with her head to one particular side, try to encourage her to move her head position, perhaps by changing toys or mobiles from side to side, or alternating the end of the cot she sleeps in, so she's got something different to look at. A rolled-up towel placed underneath her mattress might help her sleep with less pressure on the flattest part of the head – but don't try to change her head position by putting towels or pillows anywhere above the mattress. Although there are special pillows on the market that are aimed at preventing and easing positional plagiocephaly and some parents have found that they help, I would advise against pillows of any sort for safety reasons.

Whatever you do to avoid or ease the symptoms of flat head syndrome, don't be tempted to stop putting your baby on her back for sleeping. Experts are in no doubt that this simple measure really does help protect against cot death.

Dr David says: An infant with a misaligned head can be a worry for parents, but positional plagiocephaly is not painful and won't affect development of the brain, or a baby's general health in any way. It's a purely cosmetic problem.

Even in severe cases, a flattened head will usually correct itself as your baby grows and she spends more time upright and moving around. Some flattening may remain indefinitely, but shouldn't be noticeable once she has more hair. Sometimes, it's linked to a condition called torticollis, which makes the muscles on one side of the neck go into spasm and will cause a baby's head to tilt permanently to one side. Usually this can be successfully treated by a physiotherapist.

Doctors tend to advise against the use of correctional helmets or bands, which are available privately and not on the NHS, as there's no evidence they work any better than the use of repositioning techniques since re-shaping usually occurs naturally, in any case. For helmets to be effective they have to be worn for at least twenty-three hours a day, and this may result in pressure sores or skin irritation.

Very rarely, an abnormally shaped head can be the result of a genetic defect known as craniosynostosis, in which the skull plates fuse together prematurely, and which can only be corrected by surgery. This condition is more likely if the abnormal shape is noticed at birth or the flattening is at the front of the head. If your doctor suspected it, they would refer you to a specialist paediatrician for further investigation.

What the netmums say

Flat head syndrome

My little man developed a flat head on his left side due to some sort of tight neck from birth. I didn't notice it myself until a physio friend of ours pointed out that he always sat in his car seat with his head to the same side. She reckoned he probably had a tight neck from being squashed in the womb and advised us to try and help this by always offering distractions like toys and chat to the other side. We did this over the course of a few months, and his head has gradually sorted itself out. I was very concerned that his head would stay flat and very odd looking, but as he's spent more time upright it's had time to adjust back. It is now pretty much completely normal. *Jo from Fleet, mum to Hannah, three, and Jacob, eight months*

Two of my children had plagiocephaly. My son, born at thirty weeks, still has a flat head, which means he has slightly misaligned eyes, ears and jaw. Unfortunately, helmet treatments weren't available then, so he had to just live with it and was teased. My daughter, who was also premature, had a flat head, and she had a helmet. The first week she had it was very hard – I didn't realise how tight they were on their heads. However, after a week she had become used to

wearing it. She wore it through the summer, and we were able to take it off for a bit if she got too hot. It made a huge difference to her head, very quickly – so much so we stopped the treatment after six months. It was very expensive, but it was worth it.
Mel from Whitstable, mum to Harrie, thirteen, Megan, eleven, and Maisie, four

My son has a very flat head on one side. This is largely down to him having a condition called torticollis, which means the muscles in his neck weren't as stretchy on one side, and he could only turn his head in one direction. It used to worry me that he'd get bullied when he started school, but he had some physio sessions when he was about seven months old and now, although his head is still slightly flat, I don't think you'd notice if you weren't looking for it. It's almost normal now, and I put that largely down to him being able to sleep however he likes. As he's not a baby any more, he chooses to sleep on his tummy!
Cassie from Brighton, mum to Max, twenty-two months

Both of my boys have had flat head syndrome, and with my youngest it's quite significant. It was the first thing one friend pointed out, but to be honest, I don't take any notice. My eldest also has some additional needs, so to me a flat head or wonky ears are the least of our worries.
Louisa from Basildon, mum to Kit, two, and Gabriel, six months

Our first son was fine, but our second son has plagiocephaly. The doctor and health visitors have said it's something that will improve when he's sitting up and moving his head more but I don't know if I believe them. My friend's son had the same and his head is still not the right shape – my friend has problems getting hats to fit him. I don't want the same to happen to my son and I don't want him to be teased. I don't like the thought of him wearing a helmet, especially through the summer months, but we are thinking about it, even though we can't afford it. It would be a few short weeks of wearing one, but could mean a lifetime for him with a better-shaped head.
Jill from Doncaster, mum to Sean, three, and Nicholas, three months

My son was five weeks premature and has a flat head on his left side, partly from birth (he was stuck in the birth canal for a while) and partly from sleeping on his back with his head to one side. I've asked several different HVs about it and all have assured me it will right itself eventually. He's just turned a year old and it's still there now, although not as bad. But it's noticeable to us, and it is a worry that it will continue to be noticeable as he gets older. If I have another baby I will sleep them on alternate sides, to avoid this happening again.
Michelle from Nottingham, mum to Liam, twelve months

We were advised to sit our youngest twin up after feeding because he had reflux, so he spent most of his time in his baby bouncer. Before we knew it, his perfect round head was flat as a table. We just hadn't realised that sort of thing could happen. Every time we mentioned it to a health professional, we were told not to worry because it wouldn't show once his hair grew. A specialist told us that with time it would 'pop' out again but would probably never be completely round again. We thought about a helmet but by then he was nearly two years old – and besides, the specialist warned us it was very expensive, could cause sores, and didn't even always work anyway. He's four now and his head is still a bit flat, but it's lots better than it was – you can only see it if you really look.
Michelle from Chadwell Heath, mum to Billy and Charlie, four

Both of my children have been very badly affected, and I took the difficult decision to treat my second child with a helmet as his was classed as very severe, and his facial features were distorted. He only wore the helmet for a short period of time due to rapid growth and it made a big difference to him. He still has a bit of a flat head at the back but nothing more than a lot of children do. My eldest child's head is still flat at one side, but it isn't as extreme as when he was a baby. He also had torticollis and couldn't move his head very well. We tried repositioning with both children but it didn't work. I think some people worry too much about their babies having a flat head when it is only a little bit flat. My children were so severely affected even the doctor had to agree that it was not classed as usual when I took the youngest one. The decision to

use helmet therapy is a very hard one to make and it is very expensive, as it has to be done privately. I'm glad that we did it though.
Helen from Lincoln, mum to Jake, four, and Connor, two

My son, who was eleven weeks premature, had plagiocephaly. He was referred to hospital, where they assured us that it would self-correct over time and now, at just turned three, you would not notice it at all.
Alixe from Stockport, mum to Madeleine, six, and Owen, three

There was nothing wrong with Tom's head when he was born but he developed a flat side that was very noticeable. It also made his forehead misshapen, and one of his ears stick out more than the other. I tried very hard to keep him from being on his back whenever he was awake, and it seemed to help. It sounds awful but I also used medical tape to tape his ear back as a baby, as his ear would bend where he laid on it and stick out even more. Three years on his head is still slightly flat on one side, but it has got a lot better and he has lots of hair to cover it. One ear still sticks out a bit more than the other but it's not too noticeable and his forehead is fine. I think there should be more awareness of this syndrome. I had no idea it could happen.
Tanya from Liverpool, mum to Tom, three

29 Should I go back to work?

Whatever you planned for whilst expecting your baby, the questions of when and how to return to work – or indeed, whether to return to work at all – are likely to require serious consideration after you've given birth. Some mums need to go back to work for the money, some need to return for the sake of their sanity. Sometimes, it's a bit of both. In any case, take time to consider every possible option before making a decision. For most mums, some kind of compromise that allows them to work *and* be with their babies as much as possible is the most desirable route. If you're returning to the same job you had before, check out your legal rights and ask about your options. Anyone who's been with an employer for more than twenty-six weeks has the right to request flexible working hours, and although employers don't have to agree to it, they do have to give it 'serious consideration'. When it comes to sorting out childcare, research your options carefully, well in advance, and vet potential daycare settings personally – it will save on guilt and anxiety if you know you've done your utmost to ensure your little one is well looked after.

Of course, you might decide to opt for being a stay-at-home mum – at least in the foreseeable future. It's likely this will also take some adjustments. Looking after children is about as hard as any job can be, and maybe you'll have to downsize or cut back to make it economically feasible. But if it's your choice, hold your head high. Sometimes it may seem that society doesn't value you as a SAHM, but you can rest assured that your baby will.

What the experts say

Crissy says: There's undoubtedly plenty to bear in mind for a stay-at-home mum looking to become a working mum, whether that point comes for you within a few months of your baby's birth, following extended maternity leave, or once your family is complete and all your children are at school. Financial pressures may leave you little choice but to return to work, or maybe you're simply seeking to pay for a better standard of living for your family, or a few extra luxuries in life. Many mums also feel that a fulfilling role outside the home, adult contact, and some time away from their child reduces their stress levels and perhaps even makes them a better parent too. But whatever your own personal reasons for going back to work, it's important to take time to reflect upon the choices available to you and also to consider how working outside of the home will affect you and your family, both practically and emotionally. Make a list of the potential pros and cons for all involved, be clear what your priorities are, and ask yourself what you hope to gain from working, and whether these are realistic and attainable goals.

Like many mums, perhaps you'll want to compromise and return to work, but on a different timescale to before, having either negotiated a new deal with your previous employers, or looked around for something completely different instead. You may want to find out about part-time, flexi-time, job-share or shift options: don't hesitate to ask your employers what the options are and check out your employment rights if you're unsure. If it's a whole new job you're seeking, be realistic about how many hours you want, or are available to work each week, and remember to factor in time spent travelling, overtime and any 'homework'.

It's a huge decision, so don't try and shoulder it alone. Liaise closely with your partner and ask what he can offer, too, in terms of flexibility and support. Thankfully these days, lots of dads are willing and able to share parenting roles, so it's always worth exploring all *his* employment options, as well. And don't forget to consider a few 'what-ifs' at this stage, too. For instance, how will you manage if you need time off work because your baby is unwell, or your childcare lets you down at the last minute?

Some mums see having a baby as an opportunity to change careers and reinvent themselves or follow a long-cherished dream, and so may choose to retrain, study, or start their own business. These things can certainly work out well for lots of mums, but if you set out on such a path, bear in mind that whilst on paper, working from home or being self-employed can seem like the ideal solution, it can also mean long hours, and require a huge amount of self-discipline and commitment. On top of this you'll need to budget for start-up, equipment and running costs and to create a suitable workspace in your home, so make sure you do your research well in advance, as you'll need to be well prepared.

When returning to work, finding the right person or people to care for your child will probably be both your primary consideration and your biggest headache, so before you make any big decisions, think carefully about what sort of childcare you're most comfortable with, as well as what's realistically affordable.

Inevitably as a working mum, you will miss out on a certain amount of time with your baby, and sadly, the occasional guilt pangs do pretty much come with the territory. If you find that your focus always seems to be on what you and/or your child is missing, take care to remind yourself precisely why you're working and take note of all the ways in which your child benefits from having a working mum, whether it's having a more secure home life with fewer money worries, or enjoying quality time with a far more contented you. In the long run, if it turns out that either or both of you are unhappy with the new arrangements you may need to rethink and consider alternative options that may suit everyone better.

What the netmums say

Back to work

When my daughter was four months old, I went to college to study travel and tourism. I had PND, and I think getting out of the house and meeting new people helped me a lot. Then, after my son was born, I started working part-time as a barmaid in the local pub when he was six months old. I'm still working there now. This helps us financially but it's also important to me from an emotional and

social viewpoint, too. I wouldn't want to work full-time right now and even if I did, I wouldn't be able to afford the childcare.
Megan from Edinburgh, mum to Carly, four, and Stuart, fourteen months

I've taken nine months' maternity leave from my job and I'm going back for two and a half days a week but, to be honest, I'm dreading it. I'm a nursery nurse and it breaks my heart to think I'll be leaving my own little girl to look after other people's children. If I could, I'd be a stay-at-home mum. But we can't afford it.
Emma from Liverpool, mum to Anna, six months

I'm going back to work, part-time, when Oscar will be five and a half months old. My other half and I work for the same charity and our boss has worked it so that we never have to be in at the same time. It makes me happier, knowing he'll either be with me or his dad.
Rachel from Lancaster, mum to Oscar, four months

After nine months' maternity leave I returned to work three days a week. During the first two months, my hubby and I used our holiday to take turns working and looking after her, to make the transition easier. She is now at nursery two days a week, and her dad works from home one day. Financially there's no gain for us in me working, as I only really earn enough to cover the nursery fees. But we have no family or friends with children around the same age who we can see regularly, and nursery is her only chance to socialise. She loves it so much there and they do so many activities that I don't think I would have done with her on a regular basis at home. I treasure the time I get to spend with her on my days off work, and I'm happy that when I'm not around, she's in good hands and having lots of fun.
Monica from Farnham, mum to Eva, fifteen months

With my eldest daughter, I went back to work part-time after six months. She spent two days a week with a childminder, and spent a day at her grandma's – the other two days were ours. Unfortunately, I was made redundant a year later (my bosses didn't

really want part-time workers), and I'm now a full-time mum. I couldn't find another part-time job, as most roles in my field are full-time. But, although it was hard, I am glad that I get to spend the time with my daughters. I've just had our second and if I was working I wouldn't be able to return anyway. She has severe reflux, so I'm glad I'm at home to look after her.
Teresa from Paddock Wood, mum to Amelie, four, and Juliette, seven months

I am more than halfway through the six months I am taking off work, and hoping to return part-time. I always said when I had a baby I didn't want other people bringing her up, so although money will be tight I have to remind myself that time is more precious than money and things. I am loving every moment of being at home with my gorgeous girl, but I also enjoy my job and appreciate the social aspect of it, so would not want to stay at home full-time. So fingers crossed, part-time will work out to be a good compromise.
Susannah from Manchester, mum to Zahra, three months

After having Isabelle I continued my job full-time, but with compressed hours so I could work four days rather than five and have a day at home with my daughter. Now that I've had my second, I'm due to go back again soon, but have also negotiated one day a week working from home. I also work some evenings and weekends, on a rota basis throughout the year. Ideally I would not work full-time, but at the moment we can't afford for me to cut my hours. We're hoping it will be an option for us in a couple of years.
Lois from Preston, mum to Isabelle, five, and Matthew, eight months

I left work four months before the birth due to pregnancy-related ill health, intending to go back when Sophie was about six months old. But when she was born I just couldn't do it. I think if you can afford to, it's wonderful to be able to spend those precious first few formative years together. We've sacrificed foreign holidays and other luxuries to live within our means, and at times it's lonely and frustrating, but I wouldn't have missed the last five years at

home with my children. Once Chloe is at school, I will find something part-time that works around school holidays.
Alexis from Camberley, mum to Sophie, four, and Chloe, two

I lost my job two days before I found out I was pregnant and after that, no one would hire me! But I'm now glad that I don't have the pressure to return to work as much as I would have before, as it means I can enjoy watching my daughter grow up and learn new things without having been at work and potentially missing it.
Amanda from Fleet, mum to Tabitha, nine months

Pre-birth, I'd really been looking forward to taking the whole year off and had even thought that I might not go back at all. But I had a baby who used to cry constantly day and night and would hardly sleep, and after six months I couldn't take any more so persuaded my mum to look after him whilst I went back to work. He's now an absolute treasure, but I did find it tough back then.
Lucy from Wokingham, mum to Archie, six

With my son, I went back to work at about seven months, when the money ran out. I initially worked full-time for two months, then went down to part-time. With my daughter, I was in a different job, working full-time, when I had her, and I went back after nine months, again because the money ran out. My husband works shifts, which makes it easier to get Daniel to school, and he helps with household chores. I get so bored at home all day! I've found it's also better for my mental health to work, as I have PND. Thankfully I work in a school, so I get good holidays and have always finished for the day by 4 p.m. I often feel guilty and it's not always easy doing the juggling, but after the last school holidays when I couldn't cope by week two, I was glad to go back. It's nice to be using my brain.
Teresa from Long Eaton, mum to Daniel, five, and Ruth, eleven months

Eve was one when I started my job, and when I had Charlie I went back after a year, working just afternoons so I had the mornings with him. Now I've got Amy, I don't think I am going back. I'm still on leave at the moment and voluntary redundancy is to be offered so I'm going to apply for that. Charlie will be going to pre-school

soon, so it will give me some one-to-one time with Amy, which she will need. I'm lucky to have that choice, I know.
Julie from Lichfield, mum to Eve, twelve, Charlie, two, and Amy, seven months

I returned to work just one day a week when my daughter was eleven months old, so really I consider myself a stay-at-home mum. I'm a primary school teacher and felt the need to do a day, as I felt that if I didn't keep my foot in the door I would never return to teaching or keep in touch with the ever-changing education system. It's a career I wish to continue, as it's rewarding and one that's fantastic when you have a family. However, I'm lucky that my mum will travel from where she lives to look after Mia for the day. I don't think I could have done it if I had to leave her with anyone else. I know I'm lucky. It must be heart-wrenching for mums who have to return to work for financial reasons.
Katie from Leek, mum to Mia, nineteen months

My first daughter was eight months old when I went back to work, but I went back for only two and a half days a week, rather than full-time. I went back after having my second daughter when she was ten months old, doing the same days and hours as before; however, we knew when we decided to have another baby that it would mean I would eventually have to give up my job as child-care costs are so high. It would actually cost me money to go to work, as all my salary was needed to pay to have two children at the childminder's – and that was before paying for petrol to get to work! I worked the three months I needed to do to keep my maternity pay, then left. I'm now a stay-at-home mum, which is good as I don't miss out on much with the kids. However, I do miss working (although not my job!), so I hope to set up my own business next year, once Maddie goes to nursery.
Marie from Basingstoke, mum to Ellie, four, and Maddie, twenty months

30 When should I start weaning?

If you're confused and worried about weaning and when exactly is the right time to start, rest assured you're not alone. Currently, official advice is the same as it's been for the last nine years: wait until your baby is about six months old, because that's when you can be sure her digestive system is mature enough to manage solids, and she'll be developmentally ready to sit up, chew and swallow food with ease. However, unofficial advice – which you may be offered by relatives, friends, fellow mums, and even by some health professionals – will often differ. And in reality, as many as half of mums make a start on solids before their baby has reached six months old. Whatever you do, remember that there are very good reasons for not weaning before four months because, before then, your baby's digestive system will not be sufficiently developed to cope. There are good reasons, too, for not procrastinating beyond six months, as after that point, your baby starts to need more nutrients than milk alone can provide.

What's key seems to be watching your baby for signs that she's definitely ready. Remember too, that *when* you start will influence the pace you then take things at from then on. So if you do start a little earlier than recommended, make sure you take things very gradually, and if you wait, aim to move to the next stage fairly soon. (For more on starting solids, see Question 39.)

What the experts say

Louise says: It's certainly a confusing area for mums – and to be honest, many health professionals find it hard keeping up with all the changing guidelines these days. Officially, the advice of the NHS, and of the government, is that 'about six months' is still the most sensible point at which to start weaning. So I continue to recommend waiting until twenty-six weeks to wean, or – to mums who feel strongly their babies cannot wait that long – I will advise going no earlier than twenty-two weeks, in other words, about five months. If you sense that your baby is going hungry before then, I'd suggest offering her whatever she seems to need in the way of extra milk – even if that means reverting to a feed at night that you'd previously dropped. And I know that's not ideal, because the last thing you want to do is get up in the night any more frequently. But in theory, once she's eating three proper meals a day a bit later down the line, she should happily drop that night feed once more. And if she doesn't, you can help her to do so with some form of sleep training (see Question 35).

My view, overall, is that it's less about reaching a specific point, in weeks or months. It's really about the individual baby's needs, and about looking at the whole picture, to work out whether or not she's ready. So, for example, if you have a big baby who no longer seems content with just milk feeds, or has taken to waking up in the night where she's previously been sleeping through, or is sitting on your lap at mealtimes and trying to take stuff off your plate, then maybe it's time to consider weaning – even if she isn't yet six months old. You might be reassured to know that all the official guidelines – including those from the Department of Health – do also give scope for some flexibility. The fact is that babies will become ready at different stages, and the reality is that some babies may be ready to wean a bit *before* six months.

What's indisputable is that four months remains the absolute earliest you should offer solids of any sort. We know from scientific research that a baby's digestive system just isn't ready before then. Equally, experts agree that you shouldn't wait any longer than six months to make a start, because after that point your baby starts to need more in the way of iron- and zinc-rich foods. Another potential problem with waiting to wean is that sometimes it can push the whole process back, so some babies of eight or nine months or more are still eating just purées when at that stage they should have moved on to lumpy textured food or finger foods. If you do start at six months, bear in mind that you can – and should – be speedy about introducing lumpy textures and soft finger foods. If you're incorporating some baby-led weaning theories into the weaning process – which many parents do these days – you'll no doubt be doing just that anyway. (For more on baby-led weaning, see Question 39.)

Maggie says: As a keen advocate of the baby-led weaning (BLW) theory, I always advise mums that six months is, typically, a good point to start the process. That's because BLW can really only work when your baby is sitting up and supporting her own head really strongly, and her digestive system and oral motor skills are sufficiently developed to cope. Of course, all babies are different, but as a general rule that won't be until she's around six months old.

If you *do* begin weaning before six months, as I know some mums do, you're probably better off sticking to a more traditional approach with purées and spoon-feeding. You could perhaps then make a switch to a more baby-led approach when you feel she's physically ready.

Dr David says: If you can, I think it's a good idea to wait for about six months to wean, as official guidance recommends. However, this is an area where research is still being carried out, and if you do choose independently to wean a little sooner than the recommended six months, you may be reassured to hear that currently there's no clear evidence that introducing solid food somewhere between four and six months – as opposed to waiting for six months – could be harmful, either in terms of an increased risk of gastro-enteritis or respiratory tract infection, or in terms of allergies.

Government and NHS guidelines stress that you should hang on until the six month point when it comes to introducing potential allergens to babies at 'high risk' of developing an allergy – generally considered to be those who suffer from severe eczema, or those with a parent or sibling with an allergy, or with eczema, or another 'atopic' condition such as hayfever or asthma. However, the latest research suggests that even these high-risk infants are no better off if their exposure to potential allergens is delayed until after six months, rather than if you make a start somewhere between four and six months – and particularly so if you're breast-feeding, which is thought to have a protective effect against the onset of some allergies. (Don't assume if you breastfeed and/or delay weaning that it will definitely offer protection against allergies developing, however, as it may not.) My primary advice, if you have a child who falls into this high-risk camp, would be to always take professional advice before offering solids, in any case.

Regardless of whether your baby is at risk of allergies, I would *definitely* caution any parent against introducing solids before four months, because until then a baby's gut is very unlikely to be ready.

If your baby was born pre-term, you'll probably be advised to wean around six months from birth, whatever stage of development she has reached. Don't make any assumptions though, as these things should all be considered individually, and do seek advice from your healthcare team when it comes to weaning.

What the netmums say

When to wean?

We planned on waiting until the six month point, but at five and a half months, while I was eating spaghetti on toast, I noticed Tabitha watching me more intently than usual. I offered her a piece of toast and she virtually bit my hand off! She now pretty much eats what we eat (and boy does she make a mess!).
Amanda from Fleet, mum to Tabitha, nine months

Isobel is breastfed, and has always been a frequent feeder, so I had a lot of people suggesting we should wean early. Even our GP said, when she was fourteen weeks, that my milk soon wouldn't be enough for her. However I was determined to wait until six months, as recommended by the World Health Organisation guidance, which I trust. I decided early on that we were going

to try baby-led weaning and by five months, Isobel seemed physically ready for it. But we held off another couple of weeks, as I wanted to get to six months. In the end it was becoming hard to keep her away from my dinner plate, so we started at twenty-four weeks!
Claire from Southampton, mum to Isobel, seven months

Harry has always been a big, hungry baby, and when he was approaching four months, the health visitor suggested weaning, as at that point he was waking up to five times a night. It took a while for him to get going, but weaning at nineteen weeks turned out to be a good decision. After a few weeks, he was waking less and less frequently for a feed. Soon it was twice a night, then once, and now he sleeps through.
Sylvia from Winchester, mum to Harry, seven months

We started solids at six months to the day, with a mixture of purées and baby-led weaning. I felt under an immense amount of pressure to start solids before then and I won't lie, it was hard work exclusively breastfeeding for that long. But I felt I was doing the right thing waiting the extra few weeks, especially as I already knew by then that he had an allergy. Even a medical professional had suggested weaning early to 'give my boobs a rest'!
Marianne from Uddingston, mum to William, twenty-two months

My health visitor recommended baby-led weaning, and we started that at six months. Some of my mummy friends went for the more traditional puréeing, and some weaned before six months. All our babies are perfect. There was pressure by others to wean my son early, especially when he started waking up more at night at four and a half months, but I just increased his formula instead. He wasn't showing all the signs of readiness that they recommend for BLW – despite my mother-in-law's insistence that he was clearly ready for food as he watched us eating. He also intently watched us doing DIY and cooking with great interest, but he wasn't ready to have a go at either of those either!
Kayla from Fife, mum to Harry, nine months

Kieran was a very hungry baby. He would finish a bottle and want more. I put him on hungry baby formula, but he still wanted more. So at four and a half months, I weaned him on to baby rice and then on to homemade purée. I started on pear and apple, and then root vegetables, either on their own, or mixed with baby rice. He loved his food and finished it all, unlike his little sister, who wasn't fussed about milk or food in the early days. However, Kieran is now the fussy one whilst Livvy is a lot more adventurous.
Natasha from Plymouth, mum to Kieran, four, and Livvy, two

We didn't start weaning Hannah until exactly six months, simply because she wasn't interested before then and seemed quite happy with milk.
Louise from Stevenage, mum to Hannah, twenty months

My daughter was a hungry baby, waking every two hours for food even on hungry baby milk! So we introduced solids at about five months, and she went straight on to mashed (rather than puréed) and finger foods. My second is clearly not ready for food yet. She sleeps through, and I've a feeling she will be six months old before we wean her.
Clair from Portsmouth, mum to Chloe, two, and Megan, four months

Erin was weaned at four months, as per the advice then. When I had my second, I was unsure about waiting until six months, but I let her guide me. She refused anything at four months, so at six months, I tried again. She was not keen on being fed or having mushed-up food so I started to give her breadsticks and banana. This worked so I bought the baby-led weaning book, abandoned previous ideas and gave her all kinds of things to eat with her fingers, including porridge and scrambled egg! My third was weaned at four months. She liked being fed, and ate most things. I don't think there is a right or wrong way. All mine have been different.
Rachel from Bristol, mum to Erin, seven, Rowena, two, and Martha, seven months

I started weaning my little girl at around five months as she had reflux and had to take a thickening medication with each milk feed. We knew from past experience with our son who also had reflux that weaning a little sooner than recommended seemed to help the sickness. We kept her on just baby rice, which she loved from the start, until she was six months.

Julia from Shrewsbury, mum to Joel, seven, and Sasha, nine months

My daughter was breastfed on demand, but was very demanding! I stuck with it, as most advice seemed to be let your baby decide for herself when she wants food. My health visitor advised me to give formula as a supplement at four months, but unfortunately she just would not take a bottle. By then, feeds were still every two hours and taking up to forty-five minutes each time, which was exhausting. In the end I started her on solids from around five months, as she really couldn't seem to wait any longer – despite pressure from a health visitor not to 'strain her poor tummy' too early. My advice is to do what feels right for your child and not be made to feel guilty. Expert opinions seem to change so much, anyway. Not so long ago, the advice was to wean at four months, and now some experts seem to be voicing doubts about the wisdom of waiting for six months.

Melissa from Exeter, mum to Natasha, six

From birth, my daughter was underweight every week, and it's always been a struggle to feed her up. At four months she was guzzling a 6–8 oz bottle every three hours, so I was advised to start weaning. We started giving her baby rice for a few days and after a few days I began making some sweet potato and carrots, which she loves. I really worry that she has been weaned so early – but then again, her being underweight always worried me, too.

Hayley from High Wycombe, mum to Celia, five months

PART FOUR: 6–12 MONTHS

31 What can I expect from teething?

Teething experiences are really variable. Some babies 'sail through' with little or no symptoms, while others have the misery of painful gums, a raised temperature, and excessive drooling – with further unfortunate side effects that include facial rash, irritability, problems feeding and sleepless nights, the last of which is particularly galling if he's previously slept through. How much your baby suffers from bout to bout may also vary – just because he suffers badly one time, doesn't mean the next lot will be a pain, too. Many parents report that diarrhoea, nappy rash and colds also seem to crop up at teething times. There's no medical evidence to link these things with teething, although there is a theory that all the extra saliva produced makes stools looser and more acidic, which would explain the runny poo and sore bottoms. What's crucial is never *assuming* these symptoms are simply down to teething. They may need checking out by a doctor.

Typically, teething starts around six months, but your baby may cut his first tooth earlier (once in a while, a baby is even born with teeth), or later than that. An early or late start is no cause for alarm, either way. The time that teething kicks off is down to a combination of genetic and other factors, and doesn't mean anything in terms of his health or development. Babies often get the lower central incisors (the two at the bottom) through first, followed by the upper central incisors, and by the time he's three, he should have his full complement of twenty baby teeth, also known as 'deciduous' or 'milk' teeth.

What the experts say

Maggie says: Although it's sometimes known as 'cutting' teeth, the gums aren't actually cut in the teething process. Instead they naturally separate, creating a path for the tooth to push through, but this can cause inflammation and significant pain or discomfort for some babies.

Sometimes a bit of distracting play or a loving cuddle can go a long way to providing relief. Massage and biting can also help – so, for instance, you could try gently rubbing a clean finger on your baby's gum, or allowing him to bite on a clean, chilled teething ring or cold wet flannel. If he's weaned and confident with finger foods, you could also offer him a piece of chilled fruit or vegetable – cucumbers are particularly good as they retain their coldness. Don't be tempted to cool a teething relief aid in the freezer, though, as it could do more harm than good. Try to wipe any excess drool gently away, to keep facial rash at bay.

There are various teething remedies available over the counter, including anaesthetic teething gels that numb the area for a while. It's vital to get one that's age-appropriate though, and to follow the dosage instructions, so read the small print or, better still, check with your pharmacist first. There are also some 'alternative' preparations, including teething powders or granules, which some parents swear by. They're homeopathic and there's no scientific evidence that they work, but there's no harm in trying – the simple act of rubbing them into the gums is probably soothing in itself. Amber necklaces, though, are a no-no in my book, as they're costly, unproven and may put a baby at risk of choking, or even strangulation.

If your baby is over three months, you can ease pain, lower temperature – and perhaps even ensure a few hours of restful sleep for everyone – by giving him the correct dose of an appropriate infant analgesic. Do be aware that teething is only likely to cause a *slightly* raised temperature, though. If it's higher than 38.5°C, it's probably unconnected and needs checking out. That also goes for symptoms such as tummy upsets, severe nappy rash, or just general misery – always consider these as individual problems, and get medical advice. Research shows that a significant number of children admitted to one hospital had symptoms that had been wrongly associated with a tooth coming through!

Don't forget to start looking after your baby's teeth as soon as they start appearing. Buy him a little toothbrush and use a tiny amount of baby toothpaste to brush them, or simply use a clean finger, or a little piece of soft cloth. Excessive or prolonged bottle habits can cause tooth decay, so it's a good idea to think about introducing your baby to a beaker as early as possible. (For more on introducing a beaker, see Question 40.)

What the netmums say

The whole tooth

Both my daughters really suffered with teething, which they both started at nearly a year old. Before a tooth came through we'd have a couple of weeks of them being grumpy and needing Anbesol liquid on their gums and Calpol before bed so they could sleep, then just before the tooth cut, a couple of days of not eating (not even ice cream) but drinking fine, and a couple of sleepless nights. Poor things, though. I'm bad enough just with toothache!
Marie from Basingstoke, mum to Ellie, four, and Maddie, twenty months

We felt every millimetre of every tooth that came through with my son. His dreadful colic stopped at ten weeks – two weeks later, teething started. (Week 11 was bliss!) He didn't sleep through the night ever until he cut his final tooth at two and a half years. His first sentence was, 'More teeth gel please,' which tells the whole story really! When he was thirteen months and in the thick of his teething, my daughter came along. She wasn't as bad except for her molars, and had no such problems with her sleeping. Anbesol liquid and teething gel on a dummy or the gums, and a dose of Calpol where necessary always helped. Also, some ear-plugs for my other half – and plenty of concealer for me, to look vaguely human in the mornings.
Lucy from Tadworth, mum to Daniel, four, and Katie, three

Elliot started teething at three months and cut two front teeth at four months. We tried everything. Teething powders helped a bit, but teething gel just slid off his gums! We gave him Calpol at night when he was really bad – he was usually a great sleeper but teething made him regularly wake in pain. I bought every teething toy going, but they were all too big or too heavy for him to hold. On a friend's recommendation I bought some linked rings that were just small enough for him to hold and to fit in our steriliser, and could be clipped on to his buggy. On top of bright red cheeks and ears, he suffered from persistent dribbling. Plastic-backed bibs worn during the day helped to catch dribbles and prevent damp clothes, and any corresponding rashes. He also got a cough and/ or a cold every time he cut a tooth. The GP said it was not connected, but we were certain it was. Lastly, we used a dummy for longer than we would have liked, but always found that this helped settle him when teething.
Salima from Manchester, mum to Elliot, four

My oldest had her first two teeth by four months, but you wouldn't even have noticed they were on their way, apart from the chewing of everything! It seems to me that cold symptoms tend to crop up at the same time. A dose of paracetamol always helped. My youngest is a different story. His teeth take forever to cut and when they're coming through he has temper tantrums, bites his sister, and is just generally a nightmare! The only thing that settles him is Ashton and Parsons teething powders – although these don't always seem to be readily available in the shops these days.
Charise from East Kilbride, mum to Tanisha, three, and Branden, two

Alex was drooling and chewing from three months, which made him wet through, but nothing cut until seven months. He suffered with the first two, then the next few were OK, but by the time he was a year old he was constantly in discomfort with it. His temperature always shot up when a tooth was coming. We offered him teething powders, Anbesol liquid and even ibuprofen at times. My daughter got her first tooth at five months. She also seems to get a lot of relief from teething toys. The only real problem teething causes is that it can put her off her bedtime milk. So we give her

Anbesol to numb the pain about ten minutes before her feed, and it's usually OK.

Gill from Leeds, mum to Alex, two, and Lottie, nine months

My daughter started with excess drool and red cheeks at about four months. We eagerly expected some teeth, and as first-time parents, felt quite excited. We waited for other signs that teeth were on their way – grumpy, wakeful nights, and lots of tears – but they never really came. At seven months we gave up looking for teeth or signs of them. The few occasions where she seemed changed, we used teething gel and teething powders and they seemed to work well. We did, however, notice her nappies were quite disgusting for a while! Then all of a sudden, two little white marks appeared on her gums. Since then, we've had no more teeth but hopefully we'll get through them as easily as we did these. The only issue we've had is the constant drooling and the teething rash.

Caroline from Manchester, mum to Natalia, ten months

Teething came early for my children, who each had their first two teeth by the time they were three months old. My daughter had no problems with teething until her very back teeth came at eighteen months. But my son, who suffers from reflux, has had terrible problems – I have no idea if it's connected or not, but the reflux always seems worse during teething. He screams in pain and is awake most of the day and night. I found that Anbesol liquid and fabric teethers seemed to help. Teething granules were useless, though – my daughter would spit them out, and my son couldn't have them, as he has a milk allergy.

Ursula from Honiton, mum to Bronwyn, four, and Dawson, thirteen months

Tabitha got her first two bottom teeth at five months, then nothing until nine months when she got her top four within the space of a fortnight. How does teething affect her? On bad days I hardly recognise my own daughter! She suffers really badly with her teeth and when they're coming through for about a week before and a week after she is incredibly clingy and irritable. Then, thankfully,

she's back to her sunny self! Oh, and she drools for England – that's always the first giveaway!
Amanda from Fleet, mum to Tabitha, nine months

I remember asking my sister about Joey's constant dribbling when he was just a month or two old. It was obviously the start of teething, but we didn't realise. He cut his first two teeth just before he was four months old – the second was while we were camping at a festival. I had no idea why he was so miserable, then suddenly the second tooth was there! As to treatment, because I didn't realise he was teething, I just thought he was hungry, and a breastfeed always calmed him down, probably because of the sucking! He was always a terrible sleeper then, and maybe that was because he was being woken up by teething pain. When he was a bit older, we relied on Calpol. We did try a natural remedy called chamomilla powder, but I'm not convinced it helped. Thank goodness the teething days are over, though!
Anna from Birmingham, mum to Joey, three

Teething was easy peasy for Bethany. At six months, she had about three days of grizzling and then a tooth came through at the bottom. At seventeen months, she's now cutting her back teeth – it makes her a bit bad-tempered but she's fine after a dose of Calpol. Thomas is a different story. He's been cutting his teeth since he was three months old – and don't we know it! Some nights he won't stop crying until we've treated him with gel, powders, and a dose of Calpol. Then he'll still wake up an hour later! He dribbles and dribbles and dribbles. Bibs and muslins are essential and I have to keep on top of it or his chin goes red raw. I just keep reminding myself it's only a few months and then it will all be better.
Ruth from Newton Abbot, mum to Bethany, seventeen months, and Thomas, five months

32 How do I know she's developing OK?

As your baby's first year progresses, she'll grow and develop rapidly. No doubt she'll impress and delight you by doing something different with every month that passes. If you're not sure what to expect and when, there's no shortage of guidance available, in books and online. Other parents you know will probably be happy to keep you in the loop, too.

It's completely natural to want to tick off all the developmental milestones when she reaches them, and to look for regular reassurance that she's progressing as she should be. However, your baby's development is something to keep a relaxed eye on, not something to fret about – and it's definitely not a race. Try not to let those natural concerns become unnecessary anxiety, or to dwell on the opinions of competitive parents who are desperate to swap details about your baby's achievements with theirs. When it comes to baby development, there's usually a huge range of scope within what's 'normal'. And even if your baby does fall outside the suggested timeframes in one or more milestones, it doesn't necessarily mean there's a problem, just a delay. She'll get there, in most cases, in her own sweet time. If you're seriously worried because your baby doesn't seem to be developing normally in some way, your health visitor or GP should be happy to put your mind at rest, so give them a call. Chances are your worries will be unfounded – but if it does turn out there's a problem, which occasionally it can, you'll have done the right thing in getting it checked out sooner rather than later.

What the experts say

Maggie says: I know how important those developmental milestones can be. Whether it's smiling, babbling, rolling over, sitting up, grasping objects, crawling, cruising or walking, it's always a moment of great pride when your baby does something significant for the first time. It's important not to get stressed about development, though. Very often, worries are unfounded, and nearly all babies reach their various milestones eventually – it's just that some do it later than others. When they get there does not reflect how well they'll do or how much they'll achieve, in any area, later in life!

Certainly, it's a good idea to address any worries with your doctor or health visitor. You should get a formal chance to do this at the second major health review that every baby is in theory offered, at some point between seven months and a year after birth, as part of the NHS Healthy Child Programme. It's a chance for your baby's general progress to be assessed, and will usually involve questions about how well she's sleeping and eating, and whether her immunisations are up to date. Although this check should be offered to you as a matter of routine, I'm afraid that in reality, with staffing pressures common, that will not always happen. You might have to be proactive and call your local Health Visiting Team to request one, if you want one. You can usually arrange to have it done either at home, or at a clinic. If in the meantime worries arise, you should be able to talk to a member of the team on the phone. Alternatively, just make an appointment with your GP – they will refer you to a specialist if they think that's necessary.

If your baby was born prematurely, you'll probably have particular concerns about your baby's development. Prem babies will typically lag behind their full-term contemporaries for a while, but will usually catch up eventually. As a general rule, you should mark your premmie's milestones from her adjusted age, in other words, when she *would* have been born if she were full-term, and not when she actually was.

Crissy says: A baby's developmental journey is more of a marathon than a sprint, and the intensity of that amazing first year can be quite an ordeal for an anxious mum. If you have concerns, do get whatever support and advice you need to reassure yourself that your baby's healthy and well – then sit back and watch with pleasure as your baby develops at her own pace. And if other competitive mums, for whom each milestone reached becomes another notch on their mothering yardstick, are getting to you, try to bear in mind there may be good psychological reasons for this maddening behaviour. Some women see having a baby as a chance to put right what was lacking in their own upbringing, but this determination to do a better job than their own parents can spill over into their relationship with other mums. Similarly, missed opportunities or a sense of disappointment in aspects of their lives can drive women to live vicariously through their offspring. And for women who gave up work to start a family, mixed feelings about their new role and a sense that they are undervalued and invisible can sometimes play a part. Stepping straight into family life from the workplace – particularly if it was male-dominated – can be a huge shock to the system. Having had to compete to survive and shout loudest to be heard in their working life, some mums, sadly, transfer this competitive philosophy into motherhood.

What the netmums say

Marking the milestones

To be honest, I couldn't have cared less whether my kids hit the textbook milestones. All children are different and I never worried if my kids walked at a certain age, said certain words or did certain things. My son was an early walker but had speech problems whilst my daughter also walked early and is a good speaker. None of these things makes a difference to how healthy, loving or talented they are. I have never, and never will, compare my kids to anyone else's.
Chelsea from Burton-on-Trent, mum to Conner, three, and Fallon, two

I can't say I worried much, although I did compare my daughter's development with other babies, as most of my friends did. I think it's quite common for parents to do this, especially first time. I also came across others who would show off about their baby's achievements! My daughter did not have a nine-to-twelve-month health review, though. We weren't allocated a health visitor due to shortage of staff in our area and I didn't know I had to take her for one.

Monica from Farnham, mum to Eva, fifteen months

I was very interested in my first baby's milestones and followed a book from the moment I found out I was pregnant. I enjoyed seeing how he was developing in my womb, and after he was born it was reassuring to know he was reaching his milestones. Kieran got his health check at eight months old, which mainly looked at his vision, hearing and movement, although I had no concerns about these areas and all was OK. I did worry about his walking though, as he hadn't shown any interest in it by twelve months. When I had my daughter, I was a lot more relaxed about milestones, as I knew she would reach them in her own time.

Natasha from Plymouth, mum to Kieran, four, and Livvy, two

Frankie first rolled over at around five months, sat up at around six months and started crawling at eight months – although he didn't crawl very much for a couple of months: he just used to make noises until someone came and got him! Oliver rolled over at three months from back to front, then from front to back at around five months, started sitting up at six months and crawling at six months, too, which I was not prepared for at all. I had to quickly make sure everything was baby safe! There's a lot of pressure regarding milestones but mainly from other competitive mums. In the long run it doesn't matter at what age they reach their various stages. It's just a very precious moment when they do.

Lisa from Peterborough, mum to Frankie, four, and Oliver, thirteen months

I worried so much over my daughter's development as a baby that in the end I had to make myself throw my books out as I was making myself ill. My younger one is now twenty months old and I have never worried about her, she's done everything pretty much

on time. Once you're on your second child everything seems so much less worrying.
Laura from Cardiff, mum to Lila, four, and Lacey, twenty months

My daughter was born two months early and so she was a bit later than average in just about everything. I didn't worry about milestones and she has got to each one eventually. At fifteen months, she is now on the verge of walking.
Lisa from Stamford, mum to Lauren, fifteen months

I have a brilliant health visitor and she has always been there – and still is – for advice, guidance and support. I had a lot of issues with my son after he had meningitis and his development fell behind by six months. I was worried to begin with, but after a while I began to believe he would catch up in his own time. Every child is different and it would be boring if they were all the same. Even though I know they all develop at different rates I am always asking friends and family what their babies are up to at the moment; it's a normal thing and it doesn't mean you are paranoid. I do look up what the development milestones are for my child's age, but only because I'm interested in what is classified as 'the norm'! My son has had all of his checks, plus extra, due to his illnesses. My daughter is due her nine-to-twelve-month check-up this month, which I'll gladly take her to. It's good to have the peace of mind.
Sharon from Bromsgrove, mum to Louis, three, and Ella, nine months

Many of my friends compare their kids and look at development as if it's a competition. I feel very vulnerable about it, as my second daughter was premature, and for her, everything is different. Her development milestones are a lot slower. I do try not to listen to my friends and I even avoid playgroups as people often comment that she's tiny for her age, which then gets me down. Deep down I know she will catch up, but in the meantime, it's difficult.
Julie from Southend, mum to Katie, three, and Isla, nine months

I signed up for regular email newsletters for both my girls, and always checked the developmental milestones as a guide to see if they were developing normally. I don't use them as a bible, but would speak to someone from my local family support services team if the girls fell behind, as I believe early intervention can really help with any delays. I suppose, having lost my own mum early, these are a point of reference for me, though you obviously need common sense too.

Emma from Worcester Park, mum to Niamh, three, and Fionnuala, eight months

I worried like mad about my son's development, partly I think because of my professional background as a teacher for special needs, and partly because he was born five weeks early. He was late with all his milestones but now he's doing really well. My daughter was also early, but she has never given me so much concern, meeting milestones bang on. Although my health visitors were supportive, we were discharged from hospital after both births when they were a week old with no follow-up whatsoever.

Kathy from Watford, mum to Jack, three, and Charlotte, two

33 Will our sex life ever be the same again?

Your sex life can take quite a while to get back to normal after having a baby – and sometimes a long while. For many women, slow physical recovery after birth, particularly if it was a difficult one, can mean that sex hurts – and often beyond the six-week point at which doctors will generally give new mums the go-ahead to have intercourse again, if they haven't already by then. Do talk to your doctor about any problems that occur when making love, such as persistent pain or dryness. Chances are, too, the sleepless nights are taking their toll, and you'd prefer not to waste a single moment in bed that could otherwise be spent catching up on some shut-eye.

Physical factors aside, there are all sorts of emotional reasons why you might not feel much like making love again during the weeks and months after birth. You may have to give yourself some extra time to get your head round these – and if your partner's keener than you are, he may just have to wait patiently until you do. Try to keep talking, and cuddling, in the meantime. Don't put pressure on yourself to try sex again until you're ready. And when you do, remember, it could be a long time before it feels quite like it used to. Most new parents have to accept that, with a reduction in sleep, opportunity and sometimes libido, they aren't really swinging from the chandeliers much any more. There's no reason why you won't again, some day soon!

What the experts say

Crissy says: Having a baby will almost certainly have repercussions for your sex life, at least in the short term, so it's important that you and your partner have realistic expectations of how long it might be before sex is back on the agenda. Some women may feel ready for sex within weeks, for others it may take months and for some even longer, and so it's quite common for new mums to find that their partners are eager to resume lovemaking rather sooner than they are themselves. While this can understandably be a rather sensitive subject for candid discussion, if you avoid the issue you run the risk of conflict or resentment developing between you and so it's best to address any mismatch of sexual desire as soon as possible. All couples are different and there is no universal benchmark to live up to when it comes to having sex for the first time after childbirth. The only right time is when you are both ready, willing and able, so don't allow yourself to be nagged into having sex for a quiet life or because you feel guilty or neglectful of your partner. Do, however, take care to let him know that you still love and find him attractive but you're just not ready for sex yet.

It takes time for your body to recover from the physical trauma of having a baby, and the nature of the birth itself, and how rested and supported you feel in the early weeks, can impact upon your libido and your readiness to begin having sex again. You'll probably be feeling swollen and sore for quite some time following a vaginal birth, especially if you've had a tear or an episiotomy. And it's important to remember that a C-section is a major abdominal operation, so you will need a good few weeks to heal. If you're breastfeeding you may have to contend with engorgement, cracked nipples, mastitis or thrush, so your breasts may be a no-go area for some time yet.

Having a baby can also cause profound changes in how your body looks, and whilst the majority of these changes will improve or be resolved over time they can nevertheless sap a woman's self-esteem and confidence. New mums are often highly self-critical of their appearance after childbirth and may consider themselves less sexually desirable or even ugly. Some women fear that their vaginas will be so altered by childbirth that their partners will be repulsed.

If you're having similar worries try using your fingers to gently check yourself over and if you're feeling bold grab a hand mirror and have a jolly good look. Chances are once the initial swelling goes down you'll be pleasantly surprised. Although your vagina is stretched during the birth it begins to shrink and retain its muscle tone within days and although it will always be larger than it was pre-birth, pelvic floor exercises can do a lot to improve matters.

If you and your partner are ready to begin having sex sooner rather than later, it's probably best to approach each sexual encounter with no expectation of it developing into full penetrative sex. Take things slowly and gently, beginning with touching and talking about sex together. Cuddles and affection may be enough at first and if things do heat up, remember mutual masturbation or a quickie can be every bit as satisfying as a marathon event. Be spontaneous. That spur-of-the-moment extra rush of energy and affection may have passed by bedtime so be prepared to sample a little afternoon delight or a tussle on the sofa. Plan ahead for the weekend and ask someone you trust to take your baby out for a while so that the two of you can relax without fear of being disturbed. If baby-free time isn't an option, wait for nap time: providing your baby is safely tucked up in his crib he'll be none the wiser.

If it takes a while longer for your sexual desire to return, remember it's important to maintain some level of physical and emotional intimacy with your partner. So no matter how grim those sleepless nights may be, remember you're in this together and it's not OK for your partner to decamp to the spare room every night. Spend as much quality couple time together as possible, cuddle up on the sofa with a movie or cook a special meal together. If his thoughts are turning to sex while yours are firmly on sleep, try to see his desire not as an unreasonable demand but as proof that no matter what, he still needs and wants you.

What the netmums say

Bedroom tales

After a C-section, we couldn't do much at all for the first eight weeks after our son was born – it was hard enough getting in and

out of the bath! But, I must admit, I did feel a little bit of pressure to have sex again from my partner. I started to think I had better pull myself together and get on with it. Billy was in his cot in our room, and I didn't like the thought of doing it when he was so near, so his brand-new painted nursery became the place we went for a bit of passion! It's definitely got better gradually, though – so much so, I ended up pregnant again, sooner than I meant to be!
Naomi from Manchester, mum to Billy, seven months

We'd like to get the chance, but both of us working full-time, shift work and extreme tiredness stops us all the time. We always make plans to 'enjoy' each other, even trying to arrange an early session so that we're not too tired, but never seem to get round to it. It's very frustrating, and we'd love to have a regular sex life again, but just don't get the chance much.
Suzie from Harrow, mum to Isla, two

After having my first daughter, she was in intensive care for a week and then we worried about her non-stop for months after. I didn't really feel much like sex and when we did do it for the first time eight weeks after the birth, I found it really hurt. After my second daughter was born it was about ten weeks, as I was scared of it hurting again – and it did. To be honest, it still hurts a bit. The doctor can't find anything physically wrong.
Chrissy from Woking, mum to Stella, four, and Amy, nineteen months

I have had three vaginal births and after the third I suffered a vaginal prolapse. It knocked my confidence more than anything ever in my life and I scoured the internet for advice and support from others. I was afraid to have sex because of it, worrying I had become misshapen or 'baggy' down there. My breasts are also very sad these days. However, pelvic floor exercises proved to be my best friend – a year on, everything is back to normal (although my boobs are still looking south!) and our sex life is as active as the children will allow. My advice is to take things slowly, and to keep some lube close by, just in case!
Rosie from Slough, mum to Tom, eleven, Lily, three, and Arthur, thirteen months

After my son's birth I had stitches and when I went to have a coil fitted, the pain was awful. This put me off sex for ages. I also had PND, which affected the way I felt, and feared getting pregnant again. I've had a miscarriage and a healthy daughter since then, but I'm still self-conscious about my body and scared of sex. It's difficult when your husband works shifts; we never seem to have time for passion. I also find it hard with a baby in the room.
Tillie from Peterborough, mum to Christopher, five, and Carly, nine months

Thanks to sickness, raging hormones, a big belly and a painful pelvis, our sex life was more or less non-existent during pregnancy. Then my beautiful baby arrived, and being a mum for the first time meant everything was such a shock – sex was the last thing on my mind. It's taken time to adjust to our new life and for my hormones to settle. But finally, things are starting to get back on track in that department – and it's great.
Libby from Doncaster, mum to Liza, three months

I had a vaginal birth and, luckily, no stitches. We had sex again four weeks after the birth – it was painful and it didn't feel the same, although my other half insisted that it did. We now have sex once a week at least – my other half would probably like it more, but I am not in the mood as often as I used to be, and we're both generally more tired.
Chloe from London, mum to Jimmy, six months

It's taken eighteen months for our sex life to really get back to normal after the birth of my third daughter. I think there were a number of barriers. Having a baby in the bedroom who could wake up at any minute wasn't fun or relaxing. And my size-sixteen body made me very self-conscious. Lack of sleep was another problem, as she was a terrible sleeper. Finally, I suppose I would have to admit I had 'let myself go' a bit. Having a baby hanging off your boob in whatever you can be bothered to sling on with your hair unbrushed and no make-up on just doesn't make you feel very sexy. But everything's better now: she sleeps in her own bed and has a good routine, and I'm a size ten again, and much happier.
Rosa from Leicester, mum to Leya, five, Janey, four, and Keira, twenty months

We got back in the habit of regular sex pretty quickly. I think we'd both had a shock at how difficult looking after a newborn was, but it seemed to bring us closer together. It wasn't crazy-wild sex, it was more loving, 'I've-really-missed-you' sex, and it was something I think we both needed to feel human again. It was also nice to know that my hubby still found me sexy after becoming a mother. Although I was a little sore, it wasn't very painful. I think sex is an important part of our relationship, and I feel better for it. However, there are times when sleep has to come before sex!

Jennifer from Bath, mum to Matthew, two

I had a pretty traumatic labour and birth and was left with very painful and infected burst stitches, so I was sore for a long time after. I was also scared of getting pregnant again, scared it was going to hurt and very self-conscious about what I looked like 'down there'. Thankfully, my fiancé couldn't have been more supportive. He never pressured and never complained. We didn't have sex until our wee one was six months old, when I finally found the strength to just bite the bullet and go for it. We eased ourselves in gradually, and it was wonderful. I had been worried that co-sleeping would have a negative effect, but it turned out to be a good thing for our sex life. Not being able to do it in our bed just made us more adventurous!

Maria from Upminster, mum to Wilf, twenty-two months

My husband has always felt sex was his right and so, in spite of various problems that I've suffered from after birth – including a tear – he's always insisted on sex as soon as possible. It was just too much pressure to fight off while I was feeling hormonal and unable to stand up for myself, so we never waited longer than a couple of days. It has always hurt for at least a few weeks, often longer. I think women should be supported to take as long as they need. If it was up to me alone it probably would have been two or three months at least.

Carly from London, mum to Marley, six, Gina, four, and Billy, eight months

Sex, what's that? I have five kids, I'm breastfeeding, and I co-sleep with the youngest. I am just not in the mood at all. Ever!
Joely from Margate, mum to Joe, five, Lara and Harry, four, Tate, three, and Zara, seven months

34 When can I stop sterilising?

If you give your baby milk in a bottle, you'll no doubt know about the importance of sterilising. Bottles and teats need to be thoroughly cleaned to remove all traces of milk, which can quickly develop bacteria that can cause some very unpleasant tummy bugs such as gastroenteritis. Even if you wash them really well, traces of milk can remain, and so putting them daily through a steam or microwave steriliser, or in a container of cold water with sterilising solution (or – if you're stuck without any of these options – by boiling in a pan of water for ten minutes) is advisable while her immune system is still developing, and most guidelines suggest that you make this routine a daily chore until she's a year old. Once she's six months old, she'll be more robust – and will no doubt be picking up a fair few germs of her own accord, in any case, so if you've got a dishwasher you can certainly start to rely on it to keep your baby's bottles safely clean from then on.

It's not considered necessary to worry about sterilising weaning equipment, dishes and cutlery – which is just as well, because you'd no doubt struggle in most cases to fit them in your steriliser. Bung those dummies through regularly, though.

What the experts say

Louise says: I would say always sterilise bottles, teats and dummies for your baby's entire first year – although I'm sure that in reality, a lot of people probably stop doing so some months before then, and I expect the majority of those babies are fine. I do think that if you've got a dishwasher, which lots of people have these days, and you put those items through a really hot cycle, that's certainly good enough after six months. If your baby has her milk in a beaker, bear in mind that these can get seriously manky too, especially the ones with the complex valves that can trap traces of milk. I don't think it's being overcautious to run these regularly through your steriliser, assuming you can fit them in, but at the very least you need to pay careful attention to washing them. Again, if you're putting them through a hot wash in your dishwasher, you've almost certainly got it covered.

I wouldn't bother sterilising weaning bowls and spoons – and for most people, it wouldn't be practical to do so these days as sterilisers tend to be made to fit bottles only. Just be sure to wash them thoroughly in very hot soapy water and dry them with a bit of kitchen roll rather than a tea towel.

It's a good idea to keep dummies as germ-free as possible and I advise parents to carry on putting these regularly through the steriliser or dishwasher for as long as their child uses one. (It's also important to replace dummies whenever they become damaged or worn, and that goes for teats, too, because when they reach that state germs can nestle in the cracks.)

I know it might seem pointless doing all this sterilising once your baby seems so robust, is moving around, and is clearly becoming familiar with all sorts of bugs, anyway. But I think it's about limiting her exposure to the worst of dirt and germs, which put her at risk of some really nasty tummy bugs, such as gastroenteritis. For the same reason, I think parents need to pay heed to basic hygiene, too – washing hands thoroughly before making up feeds, keeping kitchen surfaces really clean, and mopping floors regularly. Personally, I also think it's a good idea to give popular toys a good clean and perhaps a dunk in some sterilising fluid occasionally, especially if you have other babies round regularly and they're having a munch on them, too. And do be very careful if you or anyone else in the house goes down with a tummy bug, as they're easily passed on. Make sure they have separate towels and that they're scrupulous about washing their hands regularly. You can't make your home sterile, of course, and neither should you, as exposure to some germs helps to build up the immune system. But it's about being sensibly clean.

What the netmums say

Keeping it clean

I was meticulous about sterilising bottles, teats and pumps for the first year as this was what was recommended by my health visitor. I used an electric steriliser, which was really easy to use, although it did take up more space than I would have liked. I didn't sterilise anything else – feeding equipment went into the dishwasher, as I was led to believe the sterilising was about the bacteria in milk, and that once babies started putting toys and other stuff in their mouths, there was no point sterilising anything else. I didn't find sterilising a chore: it was just routine, so the only relief I felt when I stopped was to have a bit more space on my kitchen counter.
Kathy from Watford, mum to Jack, three, and Charlotte, two

With my first daughter, I did everything by the book and sterilised everything – bottles, dummies, bowls and spoons, until she was twelve months old. With my second, I sterilised dummies when she was newborn only, and stopped sterilising bottles when she was about ten months old. By the time I had my son I only sterilised dummies when he was newborn and his bottles until he was about six months before giving up. Talk about getting more and more relaxed with each one!
Wendy from Cardiff, mum to Jasmine, nine, Abigail, six, and Sam, three

The few times I needed to sterilise (the odd time I expressed, and the couple of times we tried feeding expressed milk from a bottle) was before six months. I used microwave sterilising bags as they take up little space, and are re-useable. Other than that, I didn't have anything to sterilise prior to six months as I was exclusively breastfeeding – and he refused to take a bottle! By six months, I saw no point in sterilising food-related stuff as he was crawling on

the floor and putting objects in his mouth to explore, which indicated he could handle non-sterilised (but washed, of course) bowls, plates and cups – especially with a gutful of 'good bacteria' from my breast milk to bolster him.
Corinne from St Albans, mum to Isaac, three

With my daughter I sterilised bottles for nine months, but stopped once she was crawling around in the garden and began to get a taste for soil! I also sterilised bowls and spoons until then. My son is prone to tummy aches as he has an allergy to cow's milk protein so I'm still sterilising his bottles. However, I've not sterilised bowls and spoons this time round.
Claire from Woodley, mum to Cassie, five, and George, ten months

I'm still sterilising. My son's bottles and pacifiers are kept in the steriliser and it only takes a second to switch it on! His plates and bowls I wash in boiling water, and I use Dettol and Milton on everything. I like to be extra vigilant because we have cats.
Lorraine from Derby, mum to Logan, fifteen months

With both girls I only sterilised bottles for expressed milk, using the microwave steam box that came with the pump. I stopped doing that when they were crawling and putting all manner of unsavoury things in their mouths. I figured if they could survive ingesting soil and the piece of week-old pasta I'd missed when sweeping the floor, they were robust enough not to need everything sterile! I may have felt differently if I'd been using formula though.
Hilary from Sheffield, mum to Isobel, five, and Caitlin, two

I sterilised bottles and expressing equipment for up to a year, in a microwave steriliser. I never found it difficult as it only took a few minutes and I liked that the steriliser stored away in the microwave. I didn't want to take the risk of making my little boy ill should I not have washed the milk out of his bottle properly. We had special anti-colic bottles with an insert in to restrict the flow of the milk, which are excellent, but they do have a lot of places for the milk to hide in. However, I didn't sterilise anything else. He was always touching either our dog or the floor before putting his hands in his

mouth anyway. I just washed everything – bowls, spoons, toys – in hot water. I've always tried not to use too many sterilising or cleaning products in the house as my husband has asthma, and because I wanted to expose my little one to lots of bugs to build up his immune system.
Claire from Northampton, mum to Daniel, twenty months

I stopped sterilising bowls and spoons and such when my daughter was six months old. I carried on sterilising the bottles and teats till she was about ten months.
Denise from Leeds, mum to Veronica-Grace, three

With my eldest son I sterilised everything up to a year, including bottles, teats, dummies, spoons and bowls. This time round I haven't bothered with bowls and spoons and stopped sterilising dummies at about four months. There's no need to worry about bottles and teats, as he's still breastfed.
Michelle from Birmingham, mum to Tyler, four, and Morgan, eleven months

For baby number one I sterilised everything until she no longer had milk. With baby number four I gave up the steriliser the day he turned nine months! He puts just about everything in his mouth anyway and I can't sterilise the whole world so I don't even bother with the bottles and cups now, although I do make sure they are meticulously cleaned. I have never sterilised plates and spoons. The food isn't going to be sterile anyway.
Stephanie from Milton Keynes, mum to Amelia, nine, Dominic, eight, Maisie, two, and Theo, nine months

My first was breastfed until she was nine months, and when I started weaning her on to solids I just made sure the spoons and bowls I used were clean and dry. I mean, I didn't sterilise my nipples, did I? I went back to work much sooner after having my son, which left me feeling a bit overwhelmed and I became a steriliser-holic! It was only when my dad's partner pointed out that they were crawling and putting their hands in their mouth anyway, that I realised that I was going overboard. So when our third came along,

I struck a happy balance and stopped sterilising once he started to crawl.

Nicki from Sandgate, mum to Erin, five, Jack, two, and Sam, twenty-two months

I hardly sterilised at all with my eldest as she refused to take a bottle and moved straight to a cup at eight months. Similarly with my middle daughter she rarely used bottles and I didn't sterilise once she drank from a cup. My youngest is seven months and drinks milk from a bottle. I stopped sterilising at six months, but the bottles are always put on a hot cycle in the dishwasher. I sterilised dummies in the early days, but never sterilised spoons and bowls.

Rachel from Bristol, mum to Erin, seven, Rowena, two, and Martha, seven months

35 Is it OK to start sleep training?

Broken nights and the ensuing exhaustion are part of the package when you first become a parent. It's absolutely normal for young babies to wake up at least once a night, usually looking for a feed, perhaps in search of comfort or company, and often purely from habit. There's not much you can do but pander to your baby's unsociable whims at first, because until he's on solids, you can't be sure he isn't waking through genuine hunger – although there are some useful steps you can take before then, such as establishing a regular bedtime routine, teaching him to self-settle, and gradually reducing night feeds. (See Question 21.) Some amenable babies will take to sleeping through of their own accord, but many continue to wake at least once a night for many months to come. The good news is that, once your baby's past six months and weaned, you can take the matter in hand if you want to, with some sleep training. So, rather than giving him that feed, or whatever else he's looking for when he wakes in the night, or when you've put him down for the evening and he won't settle, you make sure he knows it's not available – and that he needs to go to sleep, instead. And as a general rule, the sooner you try it once he's ready, the easier it's likely to be.

Sleep training isn't for everyone. Some people prefer to let their baby lead the way and are happy to wait until he sleeps through in his own time. But not all parents can wait that long. And although sleep training can be tough, those who make a success of it tend to agree that once a whole night's sleep is on the agenda, life is a lot better. Due to space restrictions, the advice here won't be comprehensive enough to see you through sleep training. There's a full outline of the main methods in *Baby Sleep Solutions*, the Netmums guide to getting a good night's sleep, and on the Netmums website, where you can get help from experts in the sleep forum.

What the experts say

Maggie says: I'd advise waiting until your baby is at least six to nine months old and well established on solids before trying sleep training. By that point, most babies should be physically able to get through the night without a feed and if they're waking, it's more likely to be due to habit rather than hunger. Your little one should also be emotionally secure enough by now to cope without you at night – as long as he's not going through a phase of separation anxiety or some other change that could cause emotional upheaval.

These days, in the light of changing research findings, I tend to recommend that parents avoid 'controlled crying' methods of sleep training, which involve leaving a baby to cry for short periods. It's an area where there's disagreement, but some experts believe the effects of the stress hormone cortisol, which is released when a baby gets upset, is harmful to the developing brain. So my feeling is – certainly where babies under the age of one are concerned – that it's better to play safe and stick with the gentler, 'no-cry' theories, which mean you stay with your baby during sleep training, so that he's always got the reassurance of your presence. These gentler methods tend to take longer – up to six weeks – and require more time and commitment, but for parents who can't bear the thought of leaving their baby to cry, or are concerned that it could be harmful, it's a happier choice. Gradual retreat, also known sometimes as gradual withdrawal, is probably the best-known gentle method. The idea is that you stay with your baby, first sitting on a chair by his cot, and then as the evenings progress, moving the chair a little further away at a time until you are at the other side of the room – and eventually, outside the room altogether. Meanwhile, you can give verbal reassurance and strokes if you want, but don't pick him up, and try to remain 'boring' and 'unavailable', so that eventually he realises that going to sleep is probably his best option! There are other variations on the theme that can work well, if you're committed enough – for instance, Tracy Hogg's pick-up/put-down method and 'the kissing game'.

Before you start any sort of sleep training, make sure the timing's right. Don't try it if there's any other major upheaval going on in your baby's life, such as you returning to work or a house move, and avoid it if your baby is poorly, or going through a phase of separation anxiety (see Question 38). If you're planning to move your baby out of your room and into a room of his own at this stage, you might prefer to do the two things in separate phases – or bite the bullet and do both at once. It's also important to make sure you've got a bedtime routine in place, so if you haven't got one, make that the first thing you do.

For *most* babies, sleep training will be successful if you can stay committed to it. And on the whole, once you've cracked it, sleep-less nights should become a thing of the past. But sometimes, babies who've begun to sleep through can take to waking again, perhaps because of illness, teething, or some other reason for being unsettled. You might have to repeat the process in the future. Fortunately, subsequent attempts are usually quicker and easier.

Louise says: It's true that there's quite a bit of debate over 'controlled crying' sleep training methods, but for now, I'm happy to recommend it for a baby over six months who is eating solids three times a day. It's vital to do it right though, so do your research carefully first. I'd advise leaving your baby to cry for no more than three to five minutes at first, before going back to check on him. Don't turn on the lights, touch him, or make eye contact but just let him know you're there with a few reassuring words and then leave. Repeat this process, lengthening the amount of time in between checks by three to five minutes. Many sleep experts consider it safe to leave a baby for up to fifteen minutes before returning with the same quiet reassurance – if you can bear to hear him crying for that long, and not all parents can. I always say it's best to go and get on with the ironing or watch some tele-vision, rather than sitting on the stairs outside his room feeling terrible. Be prepared to go through the process repeatedly, as it's likely to take up to a week or perhaps two before the habit is broken and your baby no longer cries for your attention, but instead settles himself back to sleep when he wakes at night.

Controlled crying certainly isn't for everyone. We did it with our daughter and it was tough, but we did crack it pretty quickly and she's slept like a dream ever since. I don't believe there has been any harm caused. If you're not 100 per cent happy with this sort of sleep training, then go for a gentler method. You need to feel absolutely confident you're doing the right thing for your baby, and for you.

Crissy says: When even the professionals can't agree on the best way to teach a baby to soothe himself to sleep, how on earth are mums supposed to know what to do for the best? If you and your partner are coping well with the lack of sleep and your baby is thriving, then you may prefer to go with the flow and play a waiting game. But if after six months or more of sleepless nights your baby's nocturnal habits have left you climbing the bedroom walls then it may well be time to introduce some form of sleep training.

Before you embark on any new routine it's really important that both you and your partner agree that sleep training is the best possible option for all concerned and also that you're both fully committed to whichever method you choose to try. When the going gets tough you're going to need unconditional support and reassurance and probably a fair amount of comforting hugs, especially during those first few stressful nights, so make absolutely sure that you're doing what is right for you and your family and not simply bowing to external pressures. Remember this is not about pleasing others: it's about taking the best possible care of your baby while making sure everyone else in the family gets as much sleep as possible. If your plan is going to succeed it's essential that once you begin any sleep training you stick to your guns and remain consistent, so it's crucial that you choose your moment carefully – when your child is in good health and not teething and when there are no major family upheavals on the horizon.

Sleep training doesn't necessarily mean leaving your baby to cry it out. You may prefer a gentler, more gradual system. There's no one-size-fits-all here and what works for one infant or parent may not suit another so there's likely to be an element of trial and error. Although controlled crying may feel like the best way forward with your first baby, having light-sleeping siblings in the house may make this less of a viable option. A well-supported stay-at-home mum may be confident she can survive the exhausting few weeks that a more gradual intervention will require, while a single mum coping alone, or a working mum faced with an early start and a long day at the office may need to turn things around more quickly. At the end of the day, sleep training has to work for the whole family.

What the netmums say

Tired of being tired

We used controlled crying with our daughter. Until that point, she insisted on being held in my arms and 'bounced' to sleep. I could be standing for over an hour bouncing her up and down in my arms. Every time I put her down she would scream blue murder, and I was exhausted. I enlisted my fiancé's support, and together we laid her down and began counting down the first minute – it felt like a lifetime! I even cried myself, but my fiancé reminded me why we were doing it. After the minute, I calmed her down by rubbing her tummy and making a 'shhh' noise before letting her cry again, for two and a half minutes. We built the crying periods up to fifteen minutes and after three sets of those she fell asleep. The next night took less time, and by the third night she didn't cry at all. It was one of the best things we have done for her as she happily goes to sleep without fuss now.
Kay from Bolton, mum to Ava, seventeen months

I didn't do sleep training as such, but when my second daughter was still waking in the night at six months, my health visitor suggested watering down her formula for the night-time feed as she was taking enough milk and food during the day, and it seemed to be a comfort thing. The theory was that we'd keep diluting the feed until eventually she wouldn't wake up as it was just water. However, this didn't work, as she was simply waking up for a bottle

of water! So we decided to let her cry for a bit to see if she went back to sleep. Three nights of letting her cry for ten minutes, and we cracked it.
Marie from Basingstoke, mum to Ellie, four, and Maddie, twenty months

We are happy to let Isobel learn to sleep in her own time. If she isn't sleeping well by the time she is approaching school age, and I think it's adversely affecting her daytime behaviour, then I will use the no-cry sleep-solution method.
Claire from Southampton, mum to Isobel, seven months

I used controlled crying with both of my children. My daughter was thirteen months when she started to sleep through after three weeks of controlled crying, and my son at twenty-one months slept through after six days of controlled crying. My children are now very good sleepers and have no problems going to sleep on their own every night. I think it's kinder to sleep train than to go on being an exhausted mum, which I certainly was.
Sally from Manchester, mum to Isobel, seven, and Isaac, three

I breastfed, cuddled and rocked my son to sleep from birth until he was about eighteen months old, by which time I had stopped the breastfeeding and he was getting too big for me to 'rock' to sleep. So I decided to try the 'pick up/put down' method. It took two nights of crying. The first night I sat next to his cot for about an hour picking him up and laying him back down then patting his back as he lay (still crying) in the cot. It did seem like the longest hour of my life but the next night it took just about fifteen minutes. After that, he gradually learnt to settle himself with his music box playing and with my gradual withdrawal from his room, without crying. I understand some parents are reluctant to 'sleep train'; however, I feel everyone needs to do what is best for their child.
Erika from Thurrock, mum to William, five

We tried controlled crying with our eldest but could never see it through, as it seemed cruel at the time. He continued to wake at least twice a night until he was three, by which time we had our second, and we were exhausted. He wouldn't nap properly in the day either. My youngest was born with medical problems and between dealing with eldest waking up, and a newborn needing twenty-four-hour care, we were desperate, and ended up paying for a sleep nanny to sort out his habitual waking. My eldest is still a bit erratic with his sleep and has a tendency to creep into our bed during the night. In retrospect, I wish we'd seen the controlled crying through. The good news is that my youngest, despite his problems, sleeps very well.

Sukhi from Harrow, mum to Harman, four, and Kiran, two

A depressed, exhausted mum who cries all the time is surely more damaging than sleep training. I am on my own a lot and a full-time parent twenty-four hours a day, and the lack of sleep was making my PND far worse. Unfortunately, neither controlled crying nor gradual withdrawal seemed to work for us at the first attempt. I used Netmums guidelines on using these methods and also talked to other mums about their experiences. In the end, we had a breakthrough at around eighteen months. We were trying controlled crying, but she kept diving headfirst out of the cot and it was getting dangerous, so we abandoned it, put her in a toddler bed and tried gradual withdrawal instead, with bedtime stories, music and a lot of reassurance. All-night sleeping did not come easily for her – but it did come, eventually.

Amey from Newbury, mum to Layla, two

My daughter co-slept with me and my partner from the moment she was born, and for months we all slept brilliantly. However, at six months old she started waking every forty-five minutes and would not settle back easily, which left us all tired and ill with lack of sleep. So we decided to research sleep-training methods. Tracy Hogg's 'pick up/put down' technique seemed the kindest. We waited until my partner had five days off from work, and started the routine, having decided we might as well remove her dummy and put her in her own cot in her own room at the same time. However, every time we went in to pick Megan up it made her more upset, so the whole night was a disaster. The next night we decided to try controlled crying, and on that first night she only

woke three times and cried for no more than thirty minutes. Two nights later, she slept through and has done ever since.
Stacey from Liverpool, mum to Megan, two

I used the 'Baby Whisperer' shush/pat technique on my daughter. Until then she was rocked or cradled to sleep, essentially using my husband and myself as sleeping props. I spent a whole week in the house, concentrating on teaching her how to get to sleep herself. It was tough but got easier with each day. After that she was putting herself to sleep no problem, with little intervention – only the occasional shush/pat from either of us. This coupled with a good bedtime routine is vital, in my eyes, for young children. She's now a great sleeper, having slept through from six months, even when we're staying in hotels or with family. The first night we're somewhere new I tend to stay with her until she sleeps and often just lie my hand on her chest or back – a form of comfort from the old shush/pat days, I suppose!
Ann from Biggleswade, mum to Hannah, three

36 When will she start crawling?

It's an exciting milestone when your baby's properly on the move for the first time, and for most babies (although by no means all), crawling is likely to be the way forward. She'll need to have gained strong head control and enough muscle strength before she can master this form of 'locomotion'. You'll see her making headway in these areas when she's lying on the floor on her tummy, and perfecting mini 'push-ups'.

As to exactly when this milestone is likely to be reached, there's huge variation. Eight to nine months is typical, but she may start to crawl as early as six or seven months, and she may not crawl until nearer her first birthday, or beyond. It may be even later than that if she's found another perfectly good way of propelling herself across a room – lots of babies develop an alternative such as 'commando-style' tummy wriggling, or bottom-shuffling. And then again, she may not bother crawling at all, going straight from sitting to pulling up, standing, cruising and walking (see Question 42). Once she is on the move, it's important to look at ways of making your home as safe as possible for her now (see Question 37).

What the experts say

Louise says: Lots of parents are keen to see their baby crawling, as it's one of the major milestones, and a sign that all's going well with her development. But it's important to remember that this is a milestone with a big range of 'normal' and the timeframe in which babies do it is broad.

You can encourage your baby to crawl by giving her lots of 'tummy time' to help those arm, leg, neck and chest muscles develop, and plenty of opportunities to practise sitting up, safely propped up with cushions until she's steady enough to do so without support. Be sure not to leave her unattended, in either case. Once she's strong enough, she might then take to propping herself up on hands and knees and rocking a little, while she gathers enough confidence to actually take off. You might find she crawls backwards first rather than forwards – she'll soon be heading in the right direction, though. Putting some toys just out of her reach, or sitting a little way away yourself can offer her motivation. Let her know she's doing well with lots of praise, and she'll go from strength to strength. If you have a baby walker or 'Bumbo' chair, make sure the time she spends in it is limited, so she has plenty of opportunities to get around. Once she's on the move, ensure she's got the room and opportunity to practise. If you put cushions and other soft obstacles round the room for her to negotiate, it will provide good exercise.

It's nothing to worry about if your baby starts crawling late, or if she has an unusual way of getting from A to B. My daughter always crawled backwards and would shuffle into walls regularly, which always frustrated her no end! It doesn't really matter how your baby moves around, but as a general rule, she should be doing so, in some way, by the time she's one. It could just be a fairly simple case of delay if she's not – in which case, she'll get there eventually – but even so, it would be a good idea to have a chat to your GP or health visitor about it at that point. Don't forget to allow extra time if your baby was born pre-term – she's very likely to hit milestones like this later than is typical.

What the netmums say

On the move

Tabitha started crawling when she was five and a half months old. Well, I say crawling – she was actually just pushing herself backwards and turning in circles. It took her until she was seven and a half

months to try to go forwards and it's only now that she can go forward confidently. She isn't too bothered, though, mainly only crawling when she wants to get to something! She first attempted to roll over for the first time around six months, although she didn't get far, and then after she managed successfully, she didn't repeat it for a month.
Amanda from Fleet, mum to Tabitha, nine months

It was funny watching Tali gearing up to crawl. She seemed to be like a racer in the starting blocks, rocking back and forth on hands and knees. We found this stage of her development really exciting and encouraged her by placing things in front of her. She was so determined, but for a while she seemed to just shuffle backwards despite her best efforts and you could tell it was frustrating for her. With practice and lots of time spent backing into corners and going nowhere, she cracked crawling forward at about eight months – much to my nephew's horror, as now she was following him everywhere! She can stand too, now, and generally leaves a trail of destruction in her wake as just about everything is in her reach. She's also starting 'bear-walking', a skill which she puts to use climbing over obstacles.
Caroline from Manchester, mum to Natalia, ten months

My son didn't really crawl. It was more of a bunny-hop/bum-shuffle style of transporting himself! He began doing that at five and a half months.
Marianne from Uddingston, mum to William, twenty-two months

Owen was late with crawling. He used to just roll all around the room to get to what he wanted so he didn't crawl properly until he was thirteen months old. We're now waiting for him to start walking, but he doesn't bother trying much because he can crawl so fast – I don't think he sees the need! He can pull himself up, 'cruise' and climb the stairs now.
Alison from Sheffield, mum to Owen, sixteen months

Hannah didn't roll over until she was around nine months, and we had to wait until she was seventeen months old for her to crawl!

We tried encouraging her, but she was so happy sitting and playing with her toys, she had no reason to want to move (and even being at nursery with other babies didn't make her want to move any quicker). They say that babies tend to put their efforts into talking and motor sensory development or walking and being physically active. Hannah has lots to say already, and through baby signing classes she can sign for most things she wants to say. So I guess you can't have everything!
Louise from Stevenage, mum to Hannah, twenty months

My eldest barely moved for the first eight months of her life, then she sat up, crawled and walked in eight weeks! She never rolled over, and even now hates being on her tummy. My younger daughter shows no signs of doing anything yet. Why should she? She's got her big sister fetching and carrying for her!
Clair from Portsmouth, mum to Chloe, two, and Megan, four months

Niamh was rolling at around at four months, and sitting up unaided just before she was five months. She was crawling at five and a half months, which I hadn't expected quite so early. It was quite sudden. She'd been on her front for a few days, just moving a little bit, then one day I decided to get down next to her and crawl away from her. She followed – and within half an hour she had mastered it and has barely stopped moving around since. She's very determined. If she wants to do something, she will.
Lauren from Milton Keynes, mum to Niamh, fifteen months

My eldest, Xander, never crawled at all, although he started walking – with a helping hand – at nine months. At eight months, Zak can crawl on his knees, pull himself up using the sofa and cruise along it, and if you take his hands he will walk. It doesn't seem any time at all since they were both newborns and they are now both so independent!
Claire from Ayr, mum to Xander, four, and Zak, eight months

It was an exciting moment when my son crawled at eleven months. I had hoped he would crawl sooner, so I tried putting toys slightly out of his reach. My daughter learned to roll over at four months

and would just roll over to get herself from one end of the room to the other, before learning to 'commando crawl' at six months.
Natasha from Plymouth, mum to Kieran, four, and Livvy, two

Up until he was thirteen months, my son didn't do anything other than sit, and some weird sort of commando crawl (one straight leg, one bent leg like a wounded soldier, and dragging along by his elbows!). Then all of a sudden, at thirteen months, he learned to crawl properly, moving from bottom to knees and back again, pulling to standing and cruising furniture. I wasn't bothered it took him that long. Children will do things in their own time and no amount of mummy-rushing or worrying will change that!
Clare from Brighton, mum to Charlie, two

37 How do we make our home safe?

As many a parent has discovered, babies can be 'all over the place' once they're mobile. Natural curiosity will propel them into any new area they can find – and that includes the bits of your home and garden that present a risk to his safety. Cupboards containing bleach and drawers that hold knives are suddenly accessible. Stairs loom like mountains. And those sharp table corners you always ignored are suddenly the perfect height for him to bang his head against.

Some near-misses, bumps and scrapes are inevitable for an infant who's developing as he should be and exploring his environment as a result. But no parent can bear the thought of serious harm coming to their little one. So it's a good idea, once your baby's close to rolling, crawling, or cruising his way into trouble, to seek out the main potential hazards in your home, and adjust them so they're as safe as they can be.

That said, there's no point in being obsessive in your 'babyproofing'. However much time and money you spend, you'll probably never make it entirely safe, and besides, you don't want to create a false sense of security that makes you complacent. Keeping a close eye on your baby is still the most important step you can take to keep him safe, and educating him about troublespots, and how to negotiate them, is a sensible idea, too. You can get more detailed information about making your home a safer place for your baby on the websites of the Child Accident Prevention Trust (CAPT), and the Royal Society for the Prevention of Accidents (RoSPA).

What the experts say

Louise says: It can be tricky working out what sort of balance to go for when it comes to 'babyproofing'. Ideally, you want to remove the main risks, at least, so you're left with a reasonable environment for your baby to explore without constantly having to hover behind him. Developing babies need plenty of freedom so it's not a good idea, for example, to put them in playpens for long periods as that could be restrictive – although playpens can certainly be useful if you need to leave him in a room for a short period and want to be confident no harm will come to him. A travel cot serves the same purpose, so you certainly don't need to spend money on both.

A lot of people assume you should turn your mind to safety once your baby's crawling, but of course it's important to bear in mind that as soon as he's rolling he's at risk (and even if your baby hasn't rolled over yet, bear in mind this skill can develop suddenly). So the first rule is to never leave a baby unattended on a bed, changing unit or other high surface, for even a second. Just pop him on the floor if you need to answer the door, for example.

Once he's truly on the move, though, there are a number of essential safety issues I'd recommend thinking about – and in most cases, it's more about awareness than installing expensive equipment. Stair gates are one item, however, that I'd advise finding the money for, as I've heard of a fair few accidents involving babies and stairs. As well as having one at the top of your stairs you should probably have one at the bottom if you've got an active, exploring baby. A stair gate over the kitchen door may be helpful too, if you'd rather keep your baby out of the kitchen altogether. If you do have him in the kitchen with you, be really vigilant: make sure there are no knives, wires, pot handles or anything else dangling over surfaces or the cooker edge. Cupboard and drawer locks are favoured by some people to keep little fingers from accessing dangerous or breakable stuff, but they can be a nuisance for adults, too, and also it's quite nice if he can help himself to unbreakable pots and pans for play, so you might just be better off keeping the dodgy stuff in storage areas that aren't within his reach. If you want him to be really safe when he's with you in the kitchen, put him in a highchair with some toys or books to keep him busy.

Trapped fingers are another common injury at home so I usually recommend some sort of door-jamming devices. And I think window locks are important, on upper storey windows. Bear in mind – as with a lot of so-called childproof devices – it may not take much imagination for an older baby to work these out, so locks with keys that you can keep out of his reach are the best bet. Just don't ever put them far away in case you need to open the window in an emergency.

Drowning, sadly, is a major risk for children. As well as paying close attention to bath safety (see Question 12), you should be ultra-vigilant if there's a pond or paddling pool around. Be aware, too, if your neighbour has one, and there's any possibility your child could go walkabouts. Poisoning is another risk to be aware of. As well as obvious dangers like rat poison, medicines and bleach, less obvious products like laundry tablets and nail polish remover can be really harmful to babies if consumed in large enough quantities, so make sure everything is either locked away or well out of reach.

Watch out for electrical goods. It sounds obvious, but irons and hair straighteners should never be left on where he could touch them. Electrical wires should also be carefully tucked away. Be aware of hot bulbs and radiators, too. Cord blinds have, I'm afraid, been known to cause fatal accidents. If you have them at all, make sure they are always looped up and tightly tied out of his reach, even when he is climbing. Wardrobes, bookshelves, free-standing units and large televisions are another common danger – always make sure they're fixed to the wall.

Alongside paying attention to these major risks at home, do make sure all the equipment your child uses daily – cot, car seat, pram, and high chair, for example – comply with safety recommendations, especially if they were second-hand.

Of course, many parents do feel it's better not to babyproof their home to the nines and would rather rely on a combination of vigilance and education to keep their baby safe from risk. I think that's a fair theory, as long as you're prepared to keep a close eye on him, and you're really consistent when it comes to educating him about the risks. We've got an open fire, but we chose not to get a guard as is usually recommended, because we thought it might just draw our daughter's attention to it. Instead we've made sure she knows the fire is a danger area, and ensured we never left her alone in the room if the fire was on. And actually, I think that it's important to educate your little one about risks in the home regardless of how many you've actually removed from the equation. A loud 'no' is the best way to do this – babies learn the meaning of this word very early on, and if you're consistent about this message, he will very soon get the right idea.

It's also worth bearing in mind that you can only ever make your own house safe. That means that when you go to someone else's, you need to check it out for dangers before letting your little one loose – and be on standby to say 'no' and steer him clear of any dangers, if necessary!

What the netmums say

Safe as houses

We put a child lock on the cleaning cupboard and put stair gates up, but that was it! We felt that we wanted our kids to learn not to just open cupboards and play with whatever was inside, as we regularly go to friends' houses who don't have children, and therefore hadn't 'babyproofed' their house. It seemed to work well, and we've never had a problem.
Marie from Basingstoke, mum to Ellie, four, and Maddie, twenty months

With our first we put safety gates up and a fridge lock and cupboard door locks. With my second, I have safety gates only. I was once told by a colleague who's a mum of four that you can't stop your toddler doing dangerous things, so it's better to teach them how to do things safely. This is the best piece of advice I have ever had. I am currently teaching my eleven-month-old how to climb the stairs!
Teresa from Long Eaton, mum to Daniel, five, and Ruth, eleven months

We put baby gates to keep our daughter away from the stairs and out of the kitchen area unsupervised, and have put cleaning materials out of reach. We've also moved quite a few breakables up from baby height and we're in the process of working out how to cover our (very tiny) pond so that she can be less closely supervised in the garden.

Jess from Sheffield, mum to Lucy, seventeen months

We had nothing until our daughter started crawling, then we put safety covers over visible plug sockets and magnetic catches on the sitting room cupboard to save her turning off the PC. We also had a baby room divider, which is like a playpen that you can open up and fix to the walls. It means she's got plenty of safe space to play in. We put a temporary one on the utility room door too, which leads to the bathroom, and a permanent one at the bottom of the stairs. When she started toilet training and needed easy access to the bathroom, we took that gate down and installed magnetic locks on the cleaning cupboard and a safety foam stop to the doors. We also installed magnetic locks on the knife drawer in the kitchen and one under the sink, and reorganised the cupboards so breakables were out of reach. She was then free to explore without fear she'd hurt herself on anything that broke. The kitchen gate was taken down when she was about two and a half, and the one on the stairs on her third birthday. I just think it's better to be safe than sorry. To this day, we've still got the socket covers, and the magnetic catches on cleaning cupboards and the knife drawer.

Sharon from Northfleet, mum to Bethany, five

I didn't plan on being a relaxed mum, but it turned out I was. We never had stair gates or cupboard catches (mainly because I can't open them myself!). I taught my son to go up and down the stairs from ten months and – touch wood – he has never had an accident on them. Being a stay-at-home mum I had the luxury of being able to follow him around and even though he did go through a stage of touching and exploring everything, I tried never to make a fuss or constantly be moving things out of reach, and he soon got over it.

Vicki from Ipswich, mum to Ben, three

We put a safety gate at the top and bottom of the stairs, and covers on the plug sockets, and window locks upstairs. Chemicals we keep on a high shelf already. And we covered our pond, by getting a local metal-working company to make up a grid that fits over the top.
Helen from the Isle of Wight, mum to Lawrence, two

All we ever used were stair gates and plug socket covers. By the time we had Sam, we had bought a gorgeous marble hearth and fire surround, so when he started crawling I used to line up cushions along the hearth just in case he banged his head!
Wendy from Cardiff, mum to Jasmine, nine, Abigail, six, and Sam, three

We didn't babyproof our house. We had a stair gate at the bottom of the stairs, but that was for the dogs. My husband is always leaving tools and bits and pieces lying around, so we made sure that our son knew what he could touch and what he couldn't. We also have a wood-burning stove and have never used a fire-guard with it. I won't list some of the other things we *don't* do, as you might think I'm irresponsible! Our son has never had an accident with something that he shouldn't have had possession of. I should also say that he has always been placid and well behaved and is not a child who puts everything in his mouth. If he'd been a different character it might have caused me to take 'baby-proofing' more seriously!
Abi from Loughborough, mum to Nathaniel, four

With my first, I kept wandering around baby equipment shops looking at the safety stuff and just couldn't bring myself to buy any of it. It all just seemed a bit over the top. My older girl learned how to get up and down everything safely after I showed her once, at about seven months, how to turn round and get off the sofa back-wards. We did have a stair gate at the top of our (very steep) stairs for a while, but it was only shut when I was otherwise engaged, or at night, in case she got up and tried tottering around in her sleeping bag. She showed no interest in electrical sockets so we barely used plug covers. Beyond that we trusted her sense of

self-preservation – in general, we found that the more she was prevented from doing something, the more desperate she became to do it and therefore took more risks. We've found with her sister that we need to protect stuff from *her*, as she's a curious kind of kid! So, plug covers were purchased, CDs went up a couple of shelves, and we used hair bobbles to keep cupboard doors closed to make sure she doesn't empty all our cereals over the kitchen floor. Some stuff is second nature. Cleaning products have always been up high in our house, for example. Kids are pretty good at keeping themselves safe. The human race wouldn't be here now without a pretty strong survival instinct!
Hilary from Sheffield, mum to Isobel, five, and Caitlin, two

We gave up on cupboard locks, as my first child was better at opening them than we were. As for a stair gate, well, we lived in a shared house so it just drove everyone mad. The flat we rented next was in an old Victorian building, with incredibly steep concrete steps outside which she soon learned to climb – there didn't seem much point in stair gating the few shallow, carpeted steps inside. We now live in another flat that also has lots of steps and my older son has learnt to climb stairs safely as a result. The most important bits (bleach and knives, for example) are just common sense, and for the rest, we taught the kids to be careful, with the word 'No!' and a tap on the hand to deter them if necessary.
Abi from Mitcham, mum to Alice, eight, Byron, five, and Phoenix, eight months

38 Why does she cry when I leave her?

If your baby seems especially clingy, or has taken to bursting into tears when you leave the room or drop her off with a carer, she's probably suffering from separation anxiety. It's a problem that commonly affects babies of between six months and a year, but very typically kicks in at eight or nine months (and can also occur sometimes in toddlerhood and later in childhood, too). In a young baby, it happens because she's entered a new developmental stage: she's become conscious of a world outside her immediate vicinity, but she doesn't know for sure if you're going to come back when you leave her, and it scares her. Beyond that, it's simply a sign that she loves you like mad and doesn't want you to leave her: a not-unreasonable reaction when her main caregiver is walking away!

A clinging baby can make a mum feel guilty, sad, or frankly irritated. Having to peel a determined pair of little arms from round your neck and impress upon her you *won't* be long, and you *will* be back, can be hard. But your little one will cope, and eventually she'll come to realise that it's OK to be without you for a while, and that just because you're going away, it doesn't mean you're not coming back. Meanwhile, try not to show that you're upset when she is, as it's likely to make things worse.

What the experts say

Crissy says: Separation anxiety most commonly arises between the ages of six and nine months, as your baby first begins to grasp the notion of object permanence. Having begun to recognise herself as a separate person in her own right, she will also be able to remember objects or people, even after they have disappeared from view. Unfortunately she can't yet understand that even though you may leave her, you will also return. So faced with imminent separation from her beloved mummy, she'll protest and resist with all her might, as she's convinced that should she let you go, you will be lost to her forever. A simple game of peek-a-boo can go some way towards helping your baby learn that people don't cease to exist just because she cannot see them and in time she will come to realise that although she feels sad when you go away you will always come back to her. It's not uncommon for babies to also experience separation anxiety at night and so this is defin-itely not a good time to embark on a sleep-training plan. Take your nightly routine at a gentle pace, don't rush her and set aside plenty of time for a cuddle, story or a lullaby.

Although in some ways it may be comforting to see how attached your baby has become to you, it can also be hugely upsetting when she cries inconsolably every time you leave the room. Mums may experience conflicting emotions, at the same time feeling guilty for leaving their baby but also resentful and overwhelmed by their baby's intense need for their constant pres-ence. Unfortunately, separation anxiety often rears its head just as mums are required to return to work following maternity leave. Leaving your baby with someone she knows well, like a family member or friend, or perhaps having a nanny or babysitter care for your child in your own home can help soften the mutual blow of separation. But if your only possible childcare option is a crèche, nursery or childminder, your baby will not only need plenty of time to get to know her new caregiver, she'll also need the chance to settle into her new environment before you leave her for the first time. If possible, phase her in over the course of a week or two, gradually reducing the length of time you stay with her and increasing your absences. Your little one will have her anxiety radar set to high so you'll need nerves of steel to stay calm and to show her that you both like and approve of this strange new person. When the time comes to part from your baby, a transitional object may help to calm her and make her feel more secure, so a favoured blanket or much-loved toy may comfort and support her in your absence, as will having familiar possessions around her like her own car seat or pram. As you leave the room, keep things simple and don't drag the process out. Settle on a simple phrase or routine that will become familiar and therefore comforting for your baby, give her a special hug and kiss and then leave.

No matter how settled your baby may seem, don't be tempted to slip out when she's not looking. Also resist the urge to keep popping back, because any anxiety you show will feed her own. If you seem relaxed and composed about leaving, it will reassure and help her become accustomed to the changes in her life more quickly. You'll probably never get used to leaving your crying baby, but most mums do find ways to cope with it over time. It may help to remember that as part of their healthy development, children need to learn how to separate from their parents and it's actually part of your job description to support her in acquiring the coping skills necessary to overcome any anxiety she feels about it.

What the netmums say

Don't leave me!

My eldest used to be beside herself when I left her at the childminder's at eight months old. Her childminder encouraged me to go as she was always OK within a couple of minutes of me leaving; however it upset me so much I used to leave, then wait the other side of the door so I could hear her stop crying (and usually start giggling). We persevered and she was OK after a couple of months. Our second daughter is extremely independent. She just walked off and played, and didn't even notice me going when I dropped her off.
Marie from Basingstoke, mum to Ellie, four, and Maddie, twenty months

Chloe suffered from separation anxiety, however I had postnatal anxiety (PNA) and I think this is why. She's slowly got better but will still only stay with certain people like my mum, my brother and my best friend. She's stopped following me around the house so much

and will play on her own. My second daughter is showing no signs of it so far. It will be interesting to see if she's affected a bit later, as I'm not suffering from PNA this time around.
Clair from Portsmouth, mum to Chloe, two, and Megan, four months

At around seven months, my son would get really upset if I left him alone. He was teething at the time and often frustrated, as he was desperate to crawl. He'll play alone for a short while now, but frequently checks I'm there. As I do bits round the flat, he's now able to come with me – it's like being followed around by a noisy, determined little puppy! He gets upset in a new situation unless he can sit on my lap and takes a lot longer than other babies to get enough confidence to get down. He's fine being left with family and when his dad gets home from work, he goes straight to him. When he's upset, though, I'm the only one he wants.
Julia from London, mum to Max, eleven months

My son has suffered separation anxiety since he was about nine months old. It can drive me demented sometimes, as I cannot go to the loo, nip upstairs or wash the dishes without him hanging on the back of me. If I dare go and do something without telling him where I am he becomes hysterical! I'm a stay-at-home mum, and I think this adds to the problem, as he's never had to be left. So when he starts saying 'don't go out', I feel guilty, and more often than not end up taking him with me. He's fine with my husband but if any of the grandparents are babysitting he's not happy about it, and lets us know! I'm not sure how to get him out of it but I know if I don't sort it soon then starting at playgroup and school will be a nightmare.
Gillian from Dunfermline, mum to Tyler, two

Both my girls went to a childminder from about one onwards, and both would cry and cling on to me, leaving me feeling really guilty. Apparently they always stopped crying five minutes after I left, unlike me, who would still be upset hours later. I never did learn to cope – so much so, I ended up going part-time at work in the end.
Sarah from Nottingham, mum to Daisy, five, and Coco, three

My son had separation anxiety from birth. I couldn't have a shower without him screaming for me. This lasted right up until recently, when he started spending more time with his grandma to get used to me having to go back to work. There was nothing I could do about it really; I just tried to comfort him and stayed as close as possible to make him feel more secure. He loves his sleepovers with his grandma now, and he's also really excited about going to pre-school next year – something I never thought would ever happen!
Mandy from Garston, mum to Joseph, two

Dylan has just entered this phase. He cries when either his dad or I leave (more when it's me, though) but we deal with it by saying goodbye, telling him that we'll be back soon and keeping smiling. We don't want him to feel abandoned if we sneak away or cause tension or negative feelings. He's also recently had a couple of screaming spells when seeing people he doesn't see much!
Heather from Stockport, mum to Dylan, nine months

My daughter was a very clingy little girl. It got so bad I couldn't go into another room or she would scream. She wouldn't even go to her dad when I had to leave for work. I drove off most days in tears and when I got to work and phoned, she would still be screaming. Thankfully, I have a fantastic friend who would have her for short periods to get her used to being without me – just for fifteen minutes at first, and we gradually increased that to longer periods. It got so much easier. Since being at nursery and school she has been a confident, happy child who always says goodbye to me with a smile on her face.
Leanne from Sheffield, mum to Jasmine, five, and Joshua, two

My little girl had separation anxiety from around ten months. Before, she never wanted me, only her daddy. It was a huge shock to me, and made my PND worse. She still stands crying at the door if I leave the room, but my husband can usually distract her. If he can't, he brings her to me for a cuddle, then takes her back out. Otherwise, I'd never get the dinner made!
Rachel from Huntingdon, mum to Ruby, thirteen months

At about six months old, my little man started to go through a phase of separation anxiety. It was really bad. At times he would not settle down for the night, and I couldn't even walk across the room after putting him down without him crying. To help him understand I wasn't going anywhere permanently, I put him in his playpen safely, left the room to go to the kitchen for a few minutes, and then came back. Every time I left, I said, 'Mummy will be back in a minute.' And then when I came back, I picked him up and gave him a cuddle. I went through this process repeatedly for weeks and it was pretty tough going, especially with a three-year-old to tend to as well. It seemed to help, because a couple of months on, he has no problems at all with me leaving him for any length of time.

Lucy from Bristol, mum to Theo, three, and Morgan, eleven months

39 How do I make a start on solids?

Weaning – the gradual process of introducing a diet of solid food that will eventually replace your baby's milk feeds – can sometimes be a fraught experience. And these days, there's definitely more than one way of doing it. Traditionally, parents have begun weaning by offering spoonfuls of thin, smooth baby rice, or finely puréed fruit and vegetables. If you're a traditionalist, if you've started weaning earlier than is recommended, or if you're simply determined to keep control of exactly what your baby's consuming, perhaps you'll take this route, like many mums before you: you'll find loads of great recipes for purées on the pages of www.netmums.com. (And don't feel bad about feeding your baby from a jar when you need to.) But there's also a newer theory on the block: baby-led weaning (BLW). It means waiting until your baby is physiologically ready to sit up at the table and feed himself a selection of normal foods. It's an approach that is gaining much popularity among parents – and increasingly has the backing of health professionals, too.

Do your research when it comes to weaning. (And this isn't a comprehensive guide: you'll need to check out a more detailed source of advice before making a start.) It may seem as though the guidelines are never-ending, but they're all there for a reason, for the sake of your baby's health. Don't tie yourself in knots trying to get it right, though, and aim for a laid-back approach. Try not to push or rush your baby into eating three solid meals a day – he'll get there eventually, and besides, it's not something you can force. Give up for a few days if things don't seem to be going well, and try again a bit later.

What the experts say

Louise says: Think of weaning as a gradual process. Solid food will be a whole new concept to your baby, so introduce him to the idea gently. Let him spend time on your lap at the table or in a high chair if he's ready, so that he can see how it's done. And once you've started, accept that you'll probably only get at most a spoonful or two down him, at first.

A lot of parents offer baby rice, which has very little calorific value and is purely about offering an alternative consistency. It's certainly very bland so perhaps that's why it's not always very popular. A little cooked, puréed parsnip, sweet potato, swede or carrot might be a more appealing alternative, and cooked apple or pear, or ripe bananas or peaches, well blended, often goes down well. These can all be thinned down with a little breast or formula milk if necessary – and in fact, cows' milk, used just for cooking, in very small quantities, should be fine. Once he's shown interest in simple single flavours, you can experiment by combining them, or offering new ones. Don't only offer your baby just fruit though, or he could end up with a very sweet tooth! Remember there are certain foods you need to steer clear of in his first year: salt is an absolute no-no, whilst sugar should be kept to a minimum. Honey, shellfish, raw eggs and unpasteurised soft cheeses are all to be avoided because of the risk of food poisoning, whilst whole nuts are a choking hazard which shouldn't be offered to children under three, and very hot or spicy foods probably won't suit him. Don't forget to swot up on all the necessary safety and hygiene guidelines, too. In particular, make sure when you're reheating your baby's food that it's piping hot all the way through, and properly cooled down before you offer it.

Getting the timing right can be helpful when it comes to trying to interest your baby in his first solids. It's not usually a good idea to try when he's *really* hungry, so you might want to offer food a short while after a milk feed. Late morning or lunchtime is often a good time to kick off, rather than tea time, when he's likely to be tired. Aim to work up to just one solid feed a day, and once he's happily established on that, expand it to include a second, and then a bit later still, a third. Chances are this process will take a number of weeks, and perhaps longer, to complete. Once you and your baby have got this first phase under your belts, it'll be time to move on and offer a wider range of foods, thicker textures and lumps, and suitable 'finger foods' such as slices of soft fruit or cooked veg and bread. Of course, if you're doing baby-led weaning, you'll be offering him food this way in any case. My thoughts on the BLW approach are generally positive: it certainly makes a lot of sense, and in many ways makes for an easier life for parents, which is never a bad thing. But I'm not convinced that all babies will take everything they need in this way – and I also think there are some really good foods, such as porridge, for instance, which are just too messy to eat by hand! So I'd advocate a route that includes the best of both worlds – perhaps you'll offer a puréed or mashed meal, fed to him yourself, for lunch, and let him select from a range of appropriate but normal foods himself for tea. Or maybe you'll combine the two during one meal, spooning in a few blended veggies but simultaneously offering him some broccoli spears which he can pick up and munch on as and when he pleases.

Not all babies take happily to weaning. If your baby isn't inter-ested, don't push it. Put the purées and spoons aside for a few days and try again. If you're really worried, seek advice, but don't get stressed out. Sometimes it just takes some babies – and their mums – a while to get weaning sussed. Unless the delay is a really significant one – and you should seek professional advice if it is – it's unlikely to compromise his wellbeing if he's still getting all his usual milk feeds, too. One thing that's worth checking, if your baby doesn't seem interested in solids after six months, is how much milk he's having. Whilst milk feeds are still important at this point, too many can affect his appetite for solid food. Now could be a good time to encourage him to drop any that are surplus to requirements.

Bear in mind that weaning can be a messy business. Try to be relaxed about this – you want your baby to learn that mealtimes should be fun and enjoyable. Just cover his clothes with a bib, and the floor with a plastic cloth, and be philosophical about any clearing up that's required!

Maggie says: Like many health professionals, I was a bit sceptical about baby-led weaning theories when I first heard about them, but I've since become convinced it's a sensible way to introduce solid food to your baby. Advocates firmly believe that it allows a baby the chance to wean gradually at his own pace, encourages a healthy attitude to mealtimes and food, and reduces the likelihood that he'll grow into a 'fussy eater' a bit later on. There's even a theory that BLW babies are less likely to suffer from obesity as children. And another great benefit, from a parent's point of view, is that it makes life a lot easier, since you dispense with purées and spoon-feeding altogether. Assuming you and the rest of the family are eating a sensible, healthy diet already, you don't need to cook for your baby separately, as he just eats appropriately sized pieces of whatever you've dished up for yourself.

If you want to try baby-led weaning, then I'd say, go ahead. But do wait until he's definitely ready – sitting up well, able to pick up food and put it in his mouth, and able to chew – which, in most cases, won't be until he's about six months old. Key to the approach is sitting your baby down to eat meals at the same time as you, and allowing him to eat as little or as much as he wants. Offer foods that are easily picked up and held – for example, chunks of soft fruit, sticks of cooked vegetables, strips of meat, boneless fish, cheese, slices of egg, fingers of bread or toast, or cooked pasta spirals – and let your baby tuck in using his fingers, regardless of how much mess he makes. Eventually, when he's got the ability, you can encourage him to use cutlery instead.

Some parents worry that there's an increased choking risk with BLW, but there's no evidence that a baby being weaned this way is more likely to choke than a baby being weaned the traditional way. Gagging is common, but this is normal – it's a natural safety mechanism that allows babies to bring up anything that's not going down. If your baby gags while eating, give him a few moments and he'll almost certainly sort the situation out himself. Another worry is that you won't have all his nutrition needs covered, in particular that iron could be lacking, but there's no reason why you can't offer iron-rich foods like eggs and meat (or veggie alternatives like tofu and pulses), and as long as breast or formula feeds are also continuing, he should be fine. In fact, it's really important to remember that whenever and however you wean, milk feeds remain your baby's most important source of nourishment until he's a year old. As weaning progresses, you'll probably find he wants less milk, but he will still need around 500–600 ml (17–21 fl oz) of formula or two to three breastfeeds daily until he's a year old. And after that, it's recommended that his diet still contains around a pint of milk a day in order to get the calcium needed for healthy teeth and bone growth, although after this age, it's fine to offer full-cream cows' milk. He doesn't have to drink all this, though: you can count milk used in cooking and on cereals, and in dairy products such as cheese and yoghurt.

It's worth noting that BLW won't be suitable for all babies. Some pre-term infants or those with special needs may not have the sufficient developmental skills needed to manage it well, in which case you'd be better off taking a more traditional approach. You can always switch to BLW a bit later on, when and if he becomes ready.

Dr David says: Food allergies (an adverse immune system response to certain food proteins) are uncommon, but it's worth being alert to any bad reactions when you start the weaning process. Allergic responses usually occur within an hour of eating – or touching – a food and may result in a variety of symptoms such as an itchy rash, sneezing, red eyes, wheezing, or swelling round the mouth and eyes. Cows' milk is the most common cause of food allergy. Other allergens are eggs, peanuts, wheat, soy, tree nuts (such as hazel or brazil nuts) and fish. Sometimes strawberries, tomatoes and citrus fruits can trigger an allergy, but this will usually be a small, localised reaction round the mouth.

Do seek immediate advice from your doctor if you suspect your baby has had an allergic reaction to a food – and take care to avoid the food again in the meantime. Any child who's had a reaction, no matter how mild, should be seen by an allergy specialist if a GP can't offer tests to confirm which food is the problem. The specialist can then give advice about introducing other foods, which should help you feel confident about continuing the weaning process. I'd strongly caution against trying to self-diagnose an allergy, or using an online or postal testing service.

And do always see your GP before removing a food from your child's diet – never do this without advice first.

Usually, allergic reactions are not serious and are easily treated and, once you know what causes the problem, avoided. But very rarely – usually where nut allergies are concerned – reactions can be severe and even life-threatening. This is known as anaphylaxis and symptoms include breathing difficulties, facial swelling, severe wheezing and collapse – don't hesitate to call an ambulance if you suspect your baby is suffering.

Perhaps the biggest risk factor for allergies is having eczema, and in fact, for any child with severe eczema, a cows' milk-free diet should be tried for four to six weeks, to see if it helps the skin – which means switching to a hypoallergenic formula, or, if your child is breastfed, a dairy-free diet for you. Other risk factors include a family history of atopy – in other words, if you, your partner, or your child's sibling has an atopic condition or allergic illness – and a previous allergic reaction. If you're worried about a possible reaction, remember that it's only likely to happen with one of the common allergens listed above, and try one food at a time initially, in small amounts.

On the whole, I'd say weaning is not something to be worried about – it's something to be enjoyed!

What the netmums say

Food, glorious food

I tried baby-led weaning with my daughter, starting at six months. At first she just played with the food and it was several months before I could actually say with confidence that she was eating and digesting it. She now eats anything and everything. I cook it all from scratch so I don't have to prepare food especially for her, and she eats what we do. She still has regular breastfeeds and eats three solid meals plus snacks. We've never spoon-fed her and she is now quite adept at using cutlery, although sometimes she just finds it easier to use her hands. She also cleans her own teeth after meals!

Annette from Ashton-under-Lyne, mum to Imogen, fifteen months

For the first two to three weeks of weaning, Henry wasn't that fussed and would barely touch the spoonfuls of baby rice I was offering. So I binned the rice, tried to stop worrying, and just went with a BLW approach instead. It's great. He soon got into it, will now try anything, and eats really well. I think you have to do what you feel is right, though, and don't have to follow every bit of advice in the books. For instance, I don't let him eat yoghurt, porridge and soup with his hands. I've always preloaded the spoon for him.
Emma from Bedford, mum to Henry, nine months

A few weeks into weaning we discovered our little girl had a bad dairy allergy when her mouth swelled and her skin blistered after a spoon or two of yoghurt. I guessed immediately it was an allergy and we took her to see the emergency doctor who prescribed Piriton. Our GP then referred us to a specialist at the hospital, where they did tests that confirmed the dairy allergy – as well as an allergy to eggs. So we now have to avoid all those products, and go back to the hospital for regular check-ups. BLW seemed to work really well for us, as she much preferred being in control, and it was easier as she could eat the same sorts of things as her brother, which means a lot less food preparation for me!
Viv from Blackpool, mum to Jack, three, and Poppy, nineteen months

After much research into baby-led weaning, in the end I went with a mix of approaches. I cooked batches of purées from the fabulous Annabel Karmel book – an early favourite was sweet potato, spinach and leek. At first I just offered food at lunchtime, within two weeks we'd moved to lunch and tea and she was up to three meals a day within five weeks. Other first foods included sweet potato, butternut squash, apple, banana and pitta bread. Within three months of weaning, Hannah was eating the same food as us, which has been great.
Louise from Stevenage, mum to Hannah, twenty months

My son was born at twenty-seven weeks, and we were advised to wean at six months from his date of birth, when developmentally he was effectively three months old! We couldn't do pure baby-led weaning, as it's not practical or proven to be safe with early

babies, so I did a combination. Thankfully, he was the easiest baby to wean. He took to everything, and managed lumps right from the beginning, which I credit to him having finger foods early on. I found weaning the easiest bit of parenting, and still love watching my son eat now!
Kylie from Bury, mum to Joseph, two

At six months, after a month of baby rice, we progressed to home-made purées that I'd cooked and frozen in little pots for ease. She first tried sweet potato and liked it instantly. I made her up some recipes from Netmums and other sites, such as butternut squash and lentils, and fish pie, which she loved straight away. At six months she was also showing an interest in my toast so we tried her with some of that – she shoved it in and managed to swallow some. Now at nine months, she's still having homemade purées but they are mashed rather than puréed, and her dinner always includes some finger food. I save time by freezing small portions of any left-overs if we have a curry or casserole to mash for her next meal. We're careful not to add salt or too many spices, and add those to our own if necessary. Our son is quite fussy now and we wonder if it was because we delayed finger foods for a long time.
Julia from Shrewsbury, mum to Joel, seven, and Sasha, nine months

My first daughter just didn't show interest in solids before seven months. Once weaned, she mostly ate finger foods but some purées too, and enjoyed it all. My second daughter was weaned at around six months, as she seemed to be keen by then, and mostly had finger foods. Both girls were given whatever we were eating and we generally enjoyed mealtimes together.
Rosemary from Pontypool, mum to Chloe, five, and Lucy, three

We started weaning at nearly six months, with a selection of purées from Annabel Karmel's purée book. My daughter has Downs Syndrome, so BLW was not really an option for us, but she took to spoon-fed purées without any great difficulty. My husband and I were both at home at that time, and he likes cooking, so we both made them, preparing batches and freezing them in ice-cube trays which we could defrost and heat, a couple of cubes at a

time, in the microwave. At first everything was bashed up smooth, but we gradually made it a bit more lumpy, and she made that transition without too much difficulty. My husband was a bit of a purist at first and would not contemplate jars, but changed his mind after we stayed with someone who did not have a freezer so we did not have much choice. We realised then how convenient they were and we continued with a mix of those and home-cooked.
Ruth from Southend, mum to Lizzie, three

Max wasn't really ready when we started weaning at five and a half months, so we waited a couple of weeks and tried again. We began with homemade purées, or jars if we were out or away. Then he stole a piece of my toast and since then has had a mix of purées and finger food. He likes to eat bread or fruit himself, but will only eat vegetables and meat as purée. He isn't interested in feeding himself with a spoon yet, so I still feed him yogurt, cereal and savoury purées. I've found weaning to be the most stressful part of having a baby, as you want them to eat well, but they often have other ideas! I have to try really hard to relax and go with the flow. Listening to music helps, and if he's being difficult I just close my eyes and take a couple of breaths. Also, my friend suggested just walking away (not too far), so that they can see that it's no big deal to you whether they eat it or not (even when it is!).
Julia from London, mum to Max, eleven months

I really struggled getting my first daughter to switch to lumps: she just flat refused, which I think was down to me giving her purées for far too long! I was dreading weaning my second because of this, so this time round I pretty much started on small lumps after a few days. At seven months she now eats pretty much anything I offer her, which has made life so much easier. I guess you're just much more chilled out with your second!
Mandy from Stockport, mum to Matilda, two, and Sukie, seven months

Lily would only eat rice (really sloppy, with no lumps) and nothing else. The health visitors were worried about her weight because it had dropped loads so they were really encouraging me to get her on solids. But she would not budge, which made me worry and get really upset. After five weeks of trying something after or before every bottle (depending on how hungry she was) she eventually started to take a bit of purée! My advice is to not worry – they will eventually get there. Easier said than done, I know, but persevere.

Stacey from Maidenhead, mum to Lily, seven months

We decided to use the BLW approach, starting by including her in all our mealtimes, with a chair that allowed her to access the table. By trying to be patient and not too concerned about how much went on the floor, I felt confident that we were getting somewhere by about eight months! So, OK, maybe it was a little slower than the traditional purée approach, but at least she now knows what real food should actually look and taste like. I think a lot of people are quite rightly concerned about the choking thing, but if a child has the dexterity to pick up an appropriate piece of food and place it in their mouth, then their swallow and gut function is mature enough to deal with it. When I looked at other children of the same age (and older) that were being spoon-fed mushed-up food I was proud of the independence that she had achieved. Baby-led, all the way.

Helen from Stoke-on-Trent, mum to Isla Rose, three, and Connie May, one month

40 When should I give her a beaker?

Drinking from a cup is an important skill for your baby to learn, since water is an important and healthy supplementary drink, and because prolonged or excessive bottle habits have various health risks, not least to the teeth.

Be prepared for it to take a while to get her head round the idea of drinking from a beaker – it's a whole new skill, after all, whether she's been used to your boob or a bottle – and let her just play with it, nibble at it or spit what's in it out, if she wants. Getting to grips with a beaker is a gradual process that can take a while and cause quite a bit of mess along the way, so be patient and be prepared to stick at it if need be, experimenting with different types along the way. It's common for babies to dig their heels in on this issue – particularly when it comes to offering milk in one. Don't despair. Some babies never do accept milk in a beaker, but can often be persuaded to drink it out of a cup or through a straw, instead.

What the experts say

Louise says: Whether you're bottle-feeding or breastfeeding, it's a good idea to introduce your baby to the concept of drinking from a beaker around the same time as you start offering solid foods. Certainly it makes sense to give it a whirl early on, so she's got plenty of time to get used to the idea. There are lots of different sorts on the market, but I think the best is the most basic and usually the cheapest – a simple lidded 'free-flow' design with two handles, no valve, and three holes in the spout. Many of those available are 'non-spill', which admittedly can save on mess, but they usually come with a valve that means your baby will have to suck to get anything out and, really, the skill you're looking for her to learn is sipping.

More than likely it will be a while until your baby gets the hang of drinking from a beaker, and you'll probably have to give her some help, and show her how it's done at first. Don't push it; just make sure there's always a beaker of water available at mealtimes, and offer it periodically during the day as a thirst-quencher, especially in hot weather. Refresh it regularly, though, rather than letting the same beakerful hang around all day.

If your baby is formula-fed, your ultimate aim is to swap bottles for beakers altogether, so she has her milk as well as water in a cup. That's because there are risks associated with too much drinking of milk from a bottle. Tooth decay is one, because sucking through a teat is a process that will leave teeth exposed to the sugars in milk for longer than sipping from a cup. (And offering juice or squash in a bottle increases that risk further, which is why it's a bad idea.) The possible effect on speech and language development is another concern because, as with dummies, if a teat is in the mouth long and often enough, it could restrict opportunities to babble and talk. Extreme bottle habits are even linked to iron deficiency – if too many milk feeds are taken at the expense of a good range of solid foods – and may hamper development generally, because if a child is toting around a bottle all day, every day, it could reduce her opportunities for other activities. Of course, all these problems relate to bottle use that's prolonged and excessive, but making the switch from bottle to beaker as early as possible should save you hassle further down the line, when you've got a determined toddler who's even more reluctant to hand her bottle over. So, once she's got to grips with drinking water from a beaker, try offering a milk feed in one, and see how things go. You might be pleasantly surprised. Sometimes, offering milk in a beaker proves an acceptable alternative if you've been looking to make a switch from breast to formula but your baby hasn't been keen to accept a bottle.

All that said, many babies just won't budge when it comes to taking milk from a beaker, even once proficient at drinking water from one. It's hardly surprising, because sucking their milk through a teat probably has a comfort association for them. Many cling very steadfastly to their bottle – particularly that last one of the day, which will usually be an accepted part of the bedtime routine. Likewise, if you've been breastfeeding and you're now trying to offer formula (or, if she's passed a year old, cows' milk) in a cup, that can be a hard sell too!

Don't push it if she's not interested. Be resilient and keep trying, but it may well be that you decide to cut your losses and give up, then try again a little later. It might be worth trying a different sort of beaker, perhaps bypassing the whole notion of a spout and offering an age-appropriate, lidless cup. There are several on the market designed with babies in mind, such as the 'Doidy' cup. Other parents have found alternatives in sports bottles – or just an ordinary cup with a straw (and a bit of help).

Accepted wisdom is that babies should have given up bottles altogether by the age of one, but as many parents will testify, it can be easier said than done, particularly when it comes to that final bottle before bed – and if you've got a happy bedtime routine sussed out, you could be forgiven for not wanting to upset it. I'd say, aim to get rid of any daytime bottles after one – by which time, if she's also having some milk in cooking and on cereal, and from other dairy products, she shouldn't need more than a bottle of milk per day, anyway – but don't worry if she's still having that bedtime bottle, as long as she's also able to drink happily from a cup (and even if that is only water). Don't let her take a bottle of milk to bed with her though, because letting her lie down whilst drinking it means the milk 'bathes' the teeth, exposing them to its sugar. Furthermore, if she needs a bottle to drop off, that's not a sleep association you want to encourage. Let her have it sitting on your knee and, ideally, aim to clean her teeth afterwards.

Don't be tempted to put anything other than water or milk in your baby's beaker. Squash or flavoured milks, even if they are marketed for her age group, are best avoided because they're high in sugar, are bad for the teeth, and will just encourage an early taste for sweet things. Fresh fruit juices, although they have some nutritional value, are high in sugar too and are better avoided in her first year. If and when you do introduce them, make sure they're diluted by ten parts water to one part juice, and offer only with meals.

What the netmums say

Cup winners

Eleanor's been drinking from an open cup (the two-handled kind) for a long time now. We started her on a 'Doidy' cup around six months and she progressed very quickly on to a first cup. Funny thing is, she will only drink water from it. Put milk in and she howls and pushes it away – and she's generally not fussy at all. She's just very recently started accepting it with the lid on, but still only with water, no matter how much she wants her milk.
Susannah from York, mum to Eleanor, fourteen months

I introduced a beaker at about seven or eight months, and Elliot didn't like it at all – he was too used to sucking on a bottle. I kept trying, but no matter how much I coaxed him, he refused to drink from it. I gave up altogether when he was about one, and he ended up drinking through a straw instead of having a beaker. He drinks out of normal cups now, but still enjoys having an occasional straw.
Jeni-Ann from Darwen, mum to Elliot, two

It took a long time for both of my eldest two to learn to use beakers – neither of them was interested before ten months, and it was longer still until any of the contents actually got into their mouths! We started with water, mainly because they would just tip the contents of the beaker down themselves with great amusement. Alice would not drink milk from a beaker, but Byron did. Whether the littlest will or not, we shall have to see!
Abi from Mitcham, mum to Alice, eight, Byron, five, and Phoenix, eight months

I breastfed my son for six months, and tried introducing a beaker after that. I think it was too late and although he would drink water from a beaker and later juice, he never accepted milk from it. Given the choice of him having no milk, or drinking from a bottle, I let him have a bottle in the morning and at bedtime until recently. He's now four and has only just accepted milkshake from a cup – but still not milk. Lesson learned! I introduced a beaker a bit earlier with my daughter, at four months. She was happy to drink anything from it, milk included, and was off her bottle altogether by nine months old.

Natasha from Plymouth, mum to Kieran, four, and Livvy, two

With my twins, I tried just about every beaker on the market, and I think that was my downfall as they just ended up confused – some required sucking in a certain way, others were free-flow. The one that we eventually got the most use from was a Tommy Tippee one. We gradually progressed to removing the lids and eventually they were happy to drink from little tumblers. With my third, I stuck with the free-flow beaker and water from six months, and then on to a 'Steadycup' at eight months. By nine months, she was happy to take all daytime drinks from a beaker, and only had her bedtime and morning milk in a bottle. By twelve months, we'd ditched the bottles for that, too.

Aimee from Chester, mum to Megan and Lauren, six, and Sophie, five

My eldest boys never used a beaker at home, although they would happily drink from one at nursery! I tried every cup on the market without success. When they eventually drank from a cup they would only drink water or juice, never milk. It took until they were about four to get them away from a bottle and teat for their milk. My youngest is six months and has no interest in a beaker yet!

Kate from Plymouth, mum to Ben, eight, Seb, five, and Harry, six months

My little one went through a phase when he first started solids of being obsessed with drinking his water, which he had in a sippy cup. Now he will still drink some, but not as much. He won't touch milk in his cup, so I'm not sure how we'll manage to get him off his bottles. At his first birthday lunch recently, we discovered he

could drink from a straw (and loved it), so I've just bought him a cup with an integrated straw and may try putting his milk in that soon, and see how we go.
Julia from London, mum to Max, eleven months

Both mine tried to drink water from a Doidy cup from early on, and they've had a free-flow beaker for water since they were about seven months. I still give them their bedtime milk in a bottle to save spills over their sleeping bags. Anna took to a beaker for her mealtime milk from around eleven months, and Jonathan started to, but then was very ill with a cold and refused point-blank. However, I've recently converted him back! My advice is to keep trying. Encourage them to take a sip, but if it doesn't work go back in a month's time and try again. And introduce a free-flow beaker of water as early as you can.
Nicola from Bristol, mum to Anna and Jonathan, seventeen months

Zak got a beaker at four months, and we used to give him water in it with every meal. Although at first most of the water was spat back out, he now drinks out of it no problem. With Xander, we used a bottle-to-cup training cup and it just prolonged the process – I think going straight to a normal beaker is better. In the end, Xander used a cup with a straw in it and, from two, just a cup.
Claire from Ayr, mum to Xander, four, and Zak, eight months

My daughter drank out of a plastic beaker from about eight months, but still insisted on having her milk in the evening in a bottle. At two, we decided enough was enough, so we called in the 'baby fairies'! Florence put all her bottles in a shiny box that the 'fairies' collected when she was asleep, and in return left her with a beaker. The first few days were hard but when she asked for her bottle, we said that the fairies needed them for younger babies. She's been fine with a beaker of milk ever since.
Rachael from Swindon, mum to Florence, three

We introduced a cup to Noah at around four months – not that he actually drank out of it! But I made sure it was always there in case he changed his mind. I weaned him at six months and went

from five bottles of milk a day to two in the space of a week, with water in a free-flow cup rather than a bottle. He drank from it but only if I held it for him – and he didn't master tipping it up until he was around nine months. We did away with bottles altogether on his first birthday, with no fuss whatsoever. He has a specific blue beaker for his milk, and he's fine with it. How easy he'll find the transition from sippy cup to big-boy cup, I do not know.
Verity from Batley, mum to Noah, thirteen months

My three were all given a lidded beaker from three or four months, sometimes with water in and sometimes just to play with. My eldest two drank water, juice and milk from a beaker during the day from around seven months and were also happy to have their night-time milk in a beaker. However, my youngest won't drink formula milk from a beaker and, as he has a dairy and soya allergy, I couldn't simply substitute it for a yoghurt or some cheese. I had to wait until he gave up formula during the day to take his day bottles away. He still now has a bottle before bed and I will let him have it for as long as he wants it – as long as he isn't still doing it when he gets to school age! My oldest gave up his night-time bottle at twelve months, and if he wanted milk before bed I gave it to him in a cup. My middle one gave up her night-time bottle at about twenty months, and still has a beaker of milk before bed.
Clare from Basingstoke, mum to Michael, sixteen, Abi, three, and DJ, eighteen months

PART FIVE: 12 MONTHS +

41 Do other mums feel this bored?

For some mums, there's simply nothing more satisfying than being at home, bringing up their baby. For many of us though, full-time motherhood is not always a bed of roses – even if we imagined it would be in our pre-baby days. If you've found yourself prey sometimes to feelings of boredom, loneliness and dissatisfaction, don't feel bad, because you're definitely not alone.

It sounds awful, and not many of us care to admit it out loud, but babies can be boring. And catering for their demands can certainly be hard graft! Often, a return to work at some level (see Question 29) will provide the outlet for company and fulfilment you might be looking for. Getting out and about in the community with your baby and striking up friendships with other mums is also a guaranteed boredom buster. (And if you're not sure where to start when it comes to finding activities and hooking up with potential buddies, look no further than the local Netmums boards for inspiration.) Meanwhile, try to remember that babies grow up fast. Whether or not you're heading back to work in the near future, remind yourself on difficult days that this precious time at home with him will be over all too soon.

What the experts say

Crissy says: While motherhood can be the most joyous and rewarding of experiences, it can also simultaneously be isolating, stressful and monotonous. Adjusting to an abrupt curtailment of your personal freedom can be difficult, and being at home full-time with your baby can be a daunting challenge, particularly if you previously worked in a job you enjoyed, or where you felt valued and successful. At times, you may even fear you're inadequate for the task. And if your partner's out at work in the day, and most of the responsibility for caring for your baby rests on your shoulders, it's easy to feel resentful and taken for granted.

Boredom and isolation can trigger a great deal of frustration and anxiety in new mums, so if you're feeling ignored or unappreciated don't bottle things up. Let your partner know what's really going on for you. When emotionally sensitive issues like these are left unaddressed they can affect your sense of self-worth and over time leave you feeling depressed, overwhelmed or out of control. Mums often fall into the trap of putting everyone else's needs above their own and neglecting themselves, so give yourself permission to feel disgruntled and hard done by; after all, your whole life has been turned upside down and you're going to need to find new ways to adjust to these changes. It's entirely unrealistic to expect to be able to focus full-time on the gains of motherhood without ever considering the losses, so give yourself a break and take time out to really think about what you miss most from your old life and then work with your partner to see if you can find ways to restore some of what's been lacking.

It's amazing what the odd lie-in, cuddle on the sofa, night out with the girls or baby-free trip to the gym or shops can do for mummy morale and hopefully you'll feel like you've managed to pull back some sense of control in your life at the same time. Shake up your routine each week so you're less likely to feel stuck in a rut and get you and your baby out of the house as much as possible, especially if you're stressing over the housework and can't switch off. If you're craving contact with other adults or a chance to stretch yourself physically or intellectually, consider taking up a new hobby, joining a yoga, exercise or evening class, mother-and-baby group or online support network. Pursuing your own interests and putting yourself first now and then doesn't make you a bad mother: a happy mum really does equal a happy baby. However, now's not the time to make a start on your sequel to *War and*

Peace! Keep your goals realistic and achievable, and make sure you can fit any activities around your baby's needs, or you'll wind up feeling even more stressed.

What the netmums say

Get me outta here!

I do feel bored and lonely when at home with my little one, sometimes. I enjoy the company of other mums, especially if their babies are around the same age, as it gives us common ground and something to chat about. I suffered with PND, and I sometimes still find it hard to motivate myself to leave the house with my son on my own, so I end up sitting indoors a lot of the time. I must say, I enjoy Charlie's company much more now that he's old enough to communicate with me.
Natasha from Uxbridge, mum to Charlie, eighteen months

My husband lives abroad, and therefore I'm alone taking care of my girls. When it was just my first, I was so carried away with the joy of having her in my life that I didn't have time to feel any other way. I basked in the fact that she loved me unconditionally and knew me better than any other person in the whole world. With my second, though, I've experienced mixed feelings. I find that I crave adult conversation. Sometimes I feel like I am losing touch from reality, as I dwell mostly in the baby world. I feel lonely, and very bored. I'm always looking around for activities or play centres for babies and toddlers, as that way I'm able to meet with other mums and their kids. Even though I enjoy chatting with my toddler, I really look forward to having friends or family over.
Viva from London, mum to Chel, two, and Chan, six months

There are many times that I feel as though I will go crazy if I don't have some adult company. I need to see people at least every other day, or I feel as though I have no life outside of my family home. At the same time, I cannot quite bring myself to leave him with a stranger so I can go back to work. It's a very strange thing!
Clare from Doncaster, mum to Connor, eighteen months

I've been a stay-at-home mum since having Adam, and prior to that I'd worked for the same company for seventeen years, in a job that I loved. I couldn't justify paying all of my salary on child-care, so I opted to stay at home. Most of the time I enjoy it, but on bad days I find the routine of looking after two children mind-numbing, if I'm perfectly honest. My husband works shifts and although they can be long, he does get good time off and is a great help when he's here. We don't have much in the way of family around, so there's no support network. I've tried a few mother-and-toddler groups but didn't enjoy them, and also tried some baby gym classes, but again, didn't think they suited me, or the kids! Most of my friends who are parents work, so a lot of the time it's me and the kids. I try to ensure we do something every day. I find the lack of adult conversation and lack of thanks the hardest things to deal with – both things I had in my job. But on the other hand it's priceless being able to have this time with my kids. I know I'll never get this time back and I'm thankful that we're in a position to allow me to do that.
Eleanor from Wishaw, mum to Kaity, four, and Adam, two

Although I love spending time with my son, I do find it tedious if we're stuck without something to do for the day. It's a bit like cabin fever! Thankfully when the weather's nice we can go for a walk, and having all my other half's family within a mile means I can easily pop out for a quick chat to distract him if he's grouchy. We're usually out and about, though. My NCT group all still get together at least once a week. We did baby massage as a group, and have now started swimming classes. We also spend Monday afternoons round each other's houses having coffee and cakes, and meet up sometimes at the Baby Cafe. Then there's our weekly music session, and gather-ings of our local rural Children's Centre under-ones group. I find that even something as simple as a wander round town or a trip to the supermarket can make me feel a bit more normal. Weekends are harder as my husband is a farmer so is always working, whilst my friends are obviously spending time with their own families. Luckily my mum's also close, so I catch up with her. I know I should make the most of this time we've got together before I go back to work.
Emma from Banbury, mum to Nathaniel, four months

I definitely get lonely. Eleanor was a colicky baby, and then when that was over I had a bad winter (I have seasonal affective disorder), with the result that I didn't really get to know any mums of children her age. We go to groups but I don't generally get a chance to talk to people as Eleanor is very active and needs me to stay close to her. And most other parents I know have gone back to work, so there's a smaller pool of people to talk to anyway. Both our parents live hundreds of miles away and don't visit very regularly, and as we moved just before she was born, I don't have friends in the area. Eleanor is getting to be very good company, but still it would be so good just to have someone I could ring up and say, 'Let's go for a coffee, I can't stand being in the house any more', but there's nobody. We just go out alone. Sometimes I'm lucky and there's someone chatty in the coffee shop (who isn't a total bore), but mostly we just sit and people-watch. It feels very isolating.
Susannah from York, mum to Eleanor, fourteen months

I was really conscious that all that time at home alone with a baby could definitely tip you over the edge, especially when you hear so much about PND these days. When I am feeling a bit bored, or lonely, there seems to be two cures for me: one is extra sleep – sadly not something I get very often – and the other is simply getting out and about. It can take a real effort but it always helps. Having dogs helps too, as they have to be walked at least once a day. Going to groups is great, although it can take some perse-verance to find one that suits you and the first time you strike up a conversation can be nerve-wracking. Seeking the company of adults can make you feel selfish, but it's totally worth it. As my other half says, a happy mummy is a better mummy.
Clare from Portsmouth, mum to Edward, three months

When I had my first baby, I didn't know anyone else with young children. I tried going to baby groups, but they can be quite exclusive at times and a bit 'cliquey'. As young babies don't do much I did feel bored and lonely at home and found myself going for walks to get out the house. Eventually I found Netmums, and made some new friends with babies, which made all the

difference. Then by the time I had my youngest, I had a good network of friends with young children and groups to attend. I wasn't bored at all second time around.
Natasha from Plymouth, mum to Kieran, four, and Livvy, two

Some days I find myself bored to tears. Being with very demanding little people who are completely self-absorbed and selfish is really hard work! Sometimes I get all misty-eyed looking back to the days when I worked and was surrounded by people to talk to, then reality kicks in, and I remember that some days at work I was bored to tears too. The difference now is that I love my 'bosses'!
Yvonne from Ayr, mum to Damien, four, and Quinn, two

I never imagined that going to Sainsbury's would be exciting, or that a baby group would be the focus of my week. We usually have people over at least once a week, and when that doesn't happen it really gets to me as it means I've had little adult conversation. I've never been socially adept anyway and now I feel like I have very little to talk about to adults, beyond the news. That's why I go on Netmums. I hate the idea that I will look back on my twenties and realise that I spent it in a cocoon! We don't live near family so babysitting is very limited. And I wish I still saw people who know me primarily as me – not people I know because my other half knows them, or because our kids know each other. When my other half says he popped into the pub on the way home just because he felt like it, I realise how much I would love to be able to take myself off for a little while, too. Recently, I've started glamming up even if I'm not doing anything, to make me feel like the person I used to be. Taking the kids to activity groups helps, because it's usually a chance to mix with other adults, too. I do evening classes as well, in topics ranging from IT to belly dancing! I don't mean to sound sorry for myself. I love being a mum more than anything else I did before.
Abi from Mitcham, mum to Alice, eight, Byron, five, and Phoenix, eight months

Yes, I do get bored and lonely, and it's taken a year of cognitive behavioural therapy after PND for me to be able to say that, as I believed that saying anything negative about being a parent meant I didn't love my kids! It can be very tedious catering to a toddler and a baby's needs every day. I find that sometimes it seems like such hard work to even get out of the house that I can't be bothered, but I do, for my toddler's sake. We go to playgroup, library group and to soft play once a week. I haven't found it easy to make friends as I'm quite shy – there's a couple of other mums I like at playgroup but I haven't dared take the next step of asking them for coffee, although I get the feeling that they're as shy as me and would probably love to! So, yes, as much as I love my babies I do find it very lonely at times – it feels so good to admit that – and I wish I had something just for me.

Gina from Nottingham, mum to Niamh, two, and Isla, three months

42 When will she start walking?

It's a magic moment indeed when your baby takes those first few wobbly steps, independent of a helping hand from you. This particular milestone means a lot to most parents – and some can't help but feel a little impatient about it. But it's also a milestone that can be met within a very wide age range. So if your baby's taking her time about walking, try not to fret. In the vast majority of cases, it will be a simple case of delay, and not an actual problem. After all, if she's proficiently getting where she needs to be in some other way, why would she bother?

Your baby will need to have mastered various other skills and gained sufficient strength in her muscles before she actually takes those first tentative steps. If she's ticked off good head control, sitting up alone, and can get herself across the room in some way either by rolling, crawling, wriggling or bum-shuffling, and if she can pull herself up, and stand, or 'cruise' the room, there's no doubt that walking will come next. However, it won't necessarily come soon, as even once she's got the physical attributes she needs, it can take a while to find the required motivation and confidence! She'll probably want to cling steadfastly to the furniture, or to your hands, while she gears up for going it alone.

What the experts say

Louise says: Don't be surprised if your baby takes her first steps and then waits a while before repeating this particular party piece, reverting back to crawling, or some other safe and reliable form of getting from A to B. It's quite common – and it can be quite a while, months even, before she's tempted to repeat the experiment. It's not really clear why, but it's probably to do with confidence.

Try to let your baby go barefoot whenever she's practising her walking inside the house. In fact, babies don't really need shoes at all unless they're walking around outdoors. Barefoot is safer as she's less likely to slip, and it's easier for her to spread her toes, which will help her balance. Try to clear the decks and let her have lots of practice time, keeping a careful eye on her in case she cruises into trouble! If she's got a walker or a door bouncer, it's a good idea to put them away once she's showing signs of walking, as they can hinder development. A good piece of equipment to invest in now is a sturdy push-along toy that she can hold on to for support. Better still if it's a cart that she can put things into and take out again – another useful developmental skill to get under her belt.

There really is a very wide spectrum of normal when it comes to starting walking, as with all those milestones. Some very early walkers set off from about ten months, but thirteen to fifteen months is closer to average, and anything up to eighteen months is quite normal. My advice, generally, would be to get some reassurance from a health professional if she's not walking after that, but certainly not to worry about it if she's moving across the room in some way, and able to bear her own weight with support. She's probably just choosing not to try – babies who are very proficient crawlers or bum-shufflers may not see the point of walking! And of course, walking either early or late is in no way an indication of how bright she is, or how well she'll do later in life.

Don't worry if your baby walks on tiptoe, at first, as this is normal. But keep an eye on it. She should gradually adapt to walking on her whole foot, but if she's doing it constantly, and it's a tendency that persists beyond eighteen months, it's a good idea to mention it to your GP. A physical problem such as tight tendons could be the cause, and continuing to walk on tiptoes can exacerbate that.

What the netmums say

Taking steps

My first daughter took her first steps at nine months old, but then didn't walk again for another six weeks. Then she suddenly walked right across the room. It was such a magical and exciting time. My second daughter took her first steps at thirteen months, but then, just like her sister, waited another six weeks before starting to walk properly at fourteen months. Waiting for Anna to walk seemed to take forever! Her sister was such an early walker, so I suppose we had expected the same, but she did it in her own time. She was a much earlier talker than her sister though. Neither of them bothered with crawling.
Jill from Poole, mum to Ellen, three, and Anna, two

Thomas didn't started walking until sixteen months, and although I knew that was still within the range of normal and didn't worry about it, I couldn't help but compare him to his big sister, who walked at nine months.
Natalie from Glasgow, mum to Katie, four, and Thomas, two

My eldest daughter did not walk without assistance until she was twenty-two months old. I was quite concerned, as all her friends were walking, but she would just collapse if you didn't hold her hands and help her. I took her to see our GP as I was so concerned, but he told me not to worry, as he didn't walk until he was twenty-two months old, either! In the end I used bribery. I stood her against a chair and sat a few steps away with a pack of chocolate buttons. Within a few hours of having done it the first time, she was running around all over the place. I suspect she could have walked earlier, but was just choosing not to.
Teresa from Paddock Wood, mum to Amelie, four, and Juliette, seven months

Having bypassed the crawling phase, Connor went straight to pulling himself up on furniture, and moving from chair to chair on wobbly legs. He walked independently for the first time just before his first birthday.
Clare from Doncaster, mum to Connor, eighteen months

Both of mine were quite late walkers, although both managed to get around perfectly well without walking! My daughter was sixteen months old when she first walked, although by then she'd been cruising for months. My husband actually saw her take her first few steps when I was at work, although he didn't tell me, and when she did walk in front of me he pretended it was the first time so I wouldn't feel bad about missing it – he only recently confessed to this! My son was seventeen months when he first walked, although he'd been rolling around the room from five months. I was never concerned about them taking their time to start walking; it was everyone else that seemed concerned. I always pointed out to people who had something to say about it that the age children start walking is *not* related to their intellect!
Eleanor from Wishaw, mum to Kaity, four, and Adam, two

Lola took her first steps two weeks shy of her first birthday. Charlie took his at ten and a half months, and Archie was nine and a half months when he started walking. With Lola, I was pleased but also a bit panicky about her hurting herself. By the time Archie started I was a bit (OK, a lot) more relaxed and just let him get on with it. I'm expecting another boy and if he follows the current pattern he'll be eight and a half months when he starts walking. Kind of hoping he'll wait a bit longer though!
Helene from Leeds, mum to Lola, five, Charlie, three, and Archie, seventeen months

Our daughter, who's determined and independent, took her first steps a few days before her first birthday. When our son's first birthday came and went, he was still shuffling across the floor. An observant and relaxed child, he first walked at fourteen months. Our third child shocked us all when at ten months, he got up and tottered around the room. But he's a very social child, and loves being near his siblings. We think he probably did it just to keep up.
Nicki from Sandgate, mum to Erin, five, Jack, two, and Sam, twenty-two months

My eldest daughter was cruising by seven months so I assumed she would be an early walker, but she didn't take her first independent step until she was sixteen months old. My younger daughter Chloe was walking steadily on her own at ten months. It just goes to show you how different children are.
Alexis from Camberley, mum to Sophie, four, and Chloe, two

Trent started pulling himself up and cruising around furniture from around ten months, although he did not take his first step until he was exactly thirteen months old. It took some encouraging, as if he fell over, he wouldn't want to walk again without help for a couple of days. We found putting his comforter a few steps away from him was all the encouragement he needed. He's now confidently walking and even running. I think it was all down to confidence. Once he knew he would be OK, and could balance on his own, he was fine.
Lara from Northampton, mum to Trent, sixteen months

Damien was fourteen months when he took his first steps, three days before our first holiday abroad. Quinn waited until he was eighteen months before taking his first steps, again just days before a family holiday. The excitement must have spurred them on!
Yvonne from Ayr, mum to Damien, four, and Quinn, two

I did worry that my daughter wasn't standing up or walking, but we saw a paediatrician just after she was two and it turned out there was no point in worrying: nothing wrong, we just had to wait. She was a bum shuffler, and apparently bum shufflers are often slow to walk. She eventually stood up at about twenty-five months, and walked at twenty-seven months.
Christine from Loughborough, mum to Georgia, three

43 How can I get a longer lie-in?

Lie-ins tend to become a thing of the past once you've become parents. It's not really surprising, as the natural pattern for most babies is to fall asleep early in the evening, and that's likely to mean a correspondingly early start in the morning, too. If you've worked hard to get a bedtime routine in place and a peaceful evening to yourselves, you may well see it as pay-off worth making – particularly on days when you have to be up, anyway. And if your baby has begun sleeping through and the rest of the night was uninterrupted, you may just feel grateful for that much, at least.

Unfortunately, some babies take the definition of early riser to painful extremes! If your little one wakes at silly o'clock, you might find he'll oblige you by going back to sleep again – although to achieve this, you may have to offer a feed or a cuddle, get up to find his dummy or turn on his mobile, or simply ignore any grumblings until he gives up and drops off. If it's so early it could justifiably be considered still night-time, and you can find the energy, perhaps you'll consider a sleep training technique at this point (see Question 35). Often, though, you'll be woken by a baby who's so bright-eyed and bushy-tailed, he's clearly not going to drop off again. In this case, once you've bought yourself whatever extra minutes you can by ignoring him for a while, or by setting him up with some toys in a safe environment, your best bet is remain philosophical, and remind yourself it's temporary. One day, no doubt, you'll be shaking your 'baby' awake in order to get him up for school!

What the experts say

Maggie says: This is a very common problem. Lots of parents want to know how they can get their little ones to sleep for a bit longer, or to drop off again once awake. Younger babies can often be persuaded back to sleep for another few hours if you give them a feed. And they will sometimes – but not always – drop off again if you bring them into bed with you. Do be aware though, if you take this route, of safe sleeping guidelines (see Question 4) – and the possibility that you're setting up a habit which may become entrenched and difficult to ditch later on. Unfortunately, though, if a baby has had his quota of sleep for the night and is quite clearly up and raring to go, you cannot make him go back to sleep!

Lots of parents swear by blackout blinds, as a very dark room can convince a baby to slumber through to a more civilised waking time. The drawback is you may end up with a baby who won't drop off without them, and some sleep experts reckon you're better off teaching him to sleep under any light conditions. It can also make things tricky when you're away from home, although you can buy black-out fabric by the yard, and can perhaps rig up something temporary with a bit of Velcro or masking tape if you need to.

You'd think you could buy yourself a later start to the day by putting your baby to bed later on – and if it suits you to do so (for instance, if you don't work, so there's no rush to be up in the morning, and you're happy to keep your baby up with you in the evenings) it's worth trying to adjust your schedule, gradually over time, to see if it helps. Don't bank on it working, though. For reasons that are unclear, many babies will still wake up early, regardless of how late they were up the night before. The same tends to go for daytime naps – deliberately cutting out or reducing his naps before he's ready to drop them is no guarantee of a bit more sleep in the morning, so you may find there's no point trying.

With an older baby, it's often possible to grab some extra snoozing time by leaving him to his own devices for a while. In fact, if you take a systematic approach to this and gradually increase the number of minutes you make him wait in the morning before going in, you might eventually be able to make a significant adjustment to his schedule. Make sure he's got some safe toys and perhaps a beaker of water nearby and you may find he plays by himself quite happily for a while in the morning. If he's in a bed or climbing out of his cot, a stair gate on his bedroom door can be a boon – just make sure his room's completely safe. And for toddlers, an alarm clock can work well – you set it for a time you feel's acceptable, and make it clear he must stay in bed, or at least in his room, until then. You can buy clocks specially marketed for this, but you can also achieve the same result with a simple timer, set to turn his lamp on at a certain time. However, you may also need that stair gate if you're struggling to keep him out of your bedroom until the designated time – or some kind of reward system in place.

Generally, though, it's really just a question of accepting this particular habit as part and parcel of parenthood, and looking for practical ways of coping. Lots of couples operate a rota system so that at least you each get a chance to stay in bed on some mornings. You can also catch up on missing sleep at the start of the night, by going to bed early. And if you do have no choice but to take a wide-awake baby downstairs disagreeably early, don't feel guilty about turning the television on and flaking out on the sofa (just be wary of actually dropping off though, and leaving him unsupervised).

Babies and toddlers do grow out of early rising. You may find things improve once your baby naturally drops his daytime napping (see Question 47), and makes up for it by sleeping a little longer in the morning. But even if you don't, he *will* gradually adjust to a more sensible schedule eventually, over time. As the cliché goes, you will inevitably find at some point that you've got the opposite problem and you're struggling to get your children *out* of bed!

What the netmums say

Wakey, wakey!

My little guy used to wake up around 6.30 a.m. most mornings until I started weaning him, after which he slept until 8.30 a.m! I found the best way to minimise early waking is making sure every light

source is blocked out at night – even the slightest gap in the blinds made him wake up, so I make sure to check them before I go to bed. Also, a good-quality nappy makes a hell of a difference. A leaky nappy first thing in the morning isn't very pleasant, nor does it give you much chance of an extra ten minutes to wake up.
Pam from Arklow, mum to Ruairí, seven months

I'm not an early riser myself, so when my daughter was little I considered any wake ups at 5 or 6 a.m. to still be the middle of the night, and treated them as such by giving her a feed and putting her down again. She'd then wake later, 8.30 or 9 a.m., and that was always the start of her day. When she did start sleeping through, it was always until about 8.30 a.m., thankfully. Of course, she now has to be up by 7 a.m. for school and we both hate it!
Casey from Guildford, mum to Evie, five

My boys wake between 6 a.m. and 7 a.m. usually, but this fits with my lifestyle so I'm more than happy for them to be awake then. I did, however, want to get them used to being in their cots awake, so regardless of when they wake I always make a point of unwrapping them (they sleep in swaddle wraps), opening their curtains, talking to them and then leaving them for a short while. They're then happy to lie in their cots for half an hour or more 'talking' to themselves. They both wake around 4 a.m. for a feed, but I treat that wakening as a night feed and keep lights low, interaction minimal and put them back down awake. They generally go back to sleep within ten minutes.
Rosie from Antrim, mum to Jack and Rylan, four months

My son sleeps through now, but wakes early, at about 6 a.m. or soon after. I can leave him in his cot for thirty minutes, max, and will then bring him in with me for a while before giving him his first bottle at about 7 a.m. If I fed him at 6 a.m. when he woke, he'd then go back to sleep until 7.30 a.m., but once I'm back at work and he's at nursery, we'll both have to be up at 6 a.m. anyway, so it's important that he's OK with an early start. And it will give us some time to spend together in the morning. We don't have blackout blinds (my theory is, he can sleep in daylight during the day, so should be able to sleep according to his needs rather than by whether it's dark or not). He usually has a little chat to himself when he wakes, before he realises that he's pooed, and that's when he screams. I guess we're destined to have him wake at that time for as long he fills his nappy then.

Jo from Scarborough, mum to Ewan, four months

It came as a bit of a shock that my son woke at 4.30 a.m. for the first few months! We tried dark curtains, keeping him awake later, and just snuggling up in bed together, but nothing worked. He just settled down on his own and gradually over time progressed to sleeping until 5.30 a.m., then 6.30 a.m., then 7.30 to 8.30 a.m. Perseverance is the key!

Marianne from Uddingston, mum to William, twenty-two months

Charlie was a good sleeper, going through from 6 p.m. to 6 a.m., but in the last few months he's started waking at 4 or 4.30 a.m! Nothing will keep him in bed or get him back to sleep, so we just start our day then. The upside is that he's flaking by 6 p.m., so it makes getting him to bed easier. Occasionally, he'll crash out on the sofa or floor and if we go out in the car he's asleep in minutes. We just accept it, and hope he will get better. I have been known to be baking cakes at 5 a.m! And we go to bed early enough to make sure we've had enough sleep. Fortunately the youngest slept through from six weeks and seems to love her sleep, so doesn't usually wake until 7 a.m., when her big sister gets up for school.

Julie from Lichfield, mum to Eve, twelve, Charlie, two, and Amy, seven months

I've found that a long nap, quite late in the day, and a late bedtime, at about 9 p.m., means that my son wakes at a decent time, around 7.30 a.m. I think if you put them to bed too early they simply wake too early, and having a nap in the afternoon will give that little extra boost to keep going until 9 p.m. I have always kept to this routine, and have always had a restful night's sleep – and a reasonable lie-in.

Jennifer from London, mum to Jack, twenty-two months

My son is an early riser – has been and always will be I think. He's woken at 6 a.m. since he slept through at three months old, and still wakes at 6 a.m. now he's six years old. I've tried everything from a late supper, blackout blinds, music, later bedtimes, earlier bedtimes, you name it. Luckily, he will now play quietly or read a book in his room until we get up at 7 a.m. Sometimes you just have to accept that they are early risers, and that's the way it is. It's clearly the time of day when he's at his best. He can often be heard singing away to himself!
Melissa from York, mum to Alex, six, and Evie, four

As a young baby, Ellen was an early riser. If she woke before 5 a.m. for a feed she'd go back to sleep, but any time after 5 a.m. and she'd be wide awake and ready to start the day. When she was a little bigger and didn't cry with hunger immediately on waking, we found we could leave her for about half an hour before getting her up. Gradually she slept a bit later, until eventually it was nearer 7 a.m. Once she went in a bed at two years old we had a night light which was timed to go off at 7 a.m. and she knew that she wasn't allowed out of bed until then even if she woke early. We still do that now and it works a treat! My son wakes any time between 6 a.m. and 7 a.m. and we leave him until as near 7 a.m. as possible. He usually lasts about thirty to forty minutes just chatting to himself before he starts to fret, at which point we get him up.
Hayley from Chudleigh, mum to Ellen, five, and William, seventeen months

My two-year-old daughter has been a 6 a.m. riser since day one. It was a shock to my system at first, but I quickly got used to it and actually enjoyed having more of the morning to ourselves. She went through a phase of 8–8.30 a.m. rises, which would have been nice, except I still woke at 6 a.m. myself! Still, I was able to enjoy a quiet cuppa. Now her baby brother is around, she tends to get up when he does, at around 5 a.m. It's tough, but I'll cope. I just console myself with the thought that one day they'll be teenagers and I won't be able to get them out of bed!
Vicky from Newport Pagnell, mum to Charlotte, two, and Thomas, one month

My daughter always used to wake around 7 a.m. when she was a baby, and these days, it's anywhere between 6 a.m. and 7 a.m. I'm a morning person anyway, so I enjoyed getting up early with her and getting the day started. My wee guy, though, has been a bit different. He slept through from ten weeks old, until 7 a.m. But then it gradually changed and, with bedtime now 7.30 p.m., he wakes up between 5 a.m. and 5.45 a.m! And it doesn't matter if he goes to bed later, he never sleeps later! I'm used to it now, but my hubby finds it impossible to get up then. I just make him change the first stinky nappy of the day, instead.
Laura from Glasgow, mum to Cara, four, and Ethan, ten months

At two, Noah still wakes up any time from 4.30 a.m. We've tried everything, but have now finally accepted he's just an early riser. I try looking at it from a positive point of view – it means I can get so much done first thing: washing on the line, the evening meal prepared, and bathroom cleaned all before 7 a.m!
Kelly from Norwich, mum to Noah, two

44 When will she start talking?

Just like walking, babies' language skills develop at very different paces. Anything between twelve and eighteen months is typical when it comes to hearing those all-important early words, but that timeframe is average – some babies will have uttered one or more real words before their first birthday, and some will wait until closer to their second.

Chances are the first words she tries will be those that are easy to say and that are used a lot around her. So 'mum-ma' and 'da-da', which are usually nothing more than babbles initially, are very likely to be among the first words to actually mean something. She probably won't get her early words quite right, which is perfectly normal. Don't correct her or make a big deal out of it when she gets it wrong, but do repeat back words and sentences as they should be, so she gets the right idea. There are loads of things you can do to encourage your baby to start talking, but the most important of all is talking to her – and listening, too.

What the experts say

Louise says: Health professionals would usually be looking for a typical toddler to have around fifty comprehensible words in their vocabulary by the age of two, so if your little one hasn't started talking by then, it's something to seek advice on. As with walking, a lack of chat beyond this 'average' timeframe may be a simple delay that is no cause for worry – if she's babbling well and doesn't seem to have a problem understanding what *you're* saying, she's probably just taking her time. Sometimes, though, a lack of chat can signal a problem, perhaps with hearing, so it's well worth getting checked out. Speech and language difficulties tend to be better tackled sooner than later, and as it can take a while for an appointment with a specialist to come through, you should certainly seek advice from your health visitor or GP whenever you become concerned – you can always cancel it if it turns out you need to. Often with a late starter, you'll find there's no stopping her once she does get talking, and she'll very soon have a great deal to say for herself.

There's no doubt that parental input is hugely significant when it comes to learning to talk, which is why it's so important to talk to your baby. It doesn't always come naturally to do so – some parents feel a bit uncomfortable about it, but it really is so vital. Rest assured she will love the sound of your voice and you never have to feel daft conversing with her. It's fine to use simple language, but try to avoid using 'baby talk'. Aim to talk normally, in a descriptive, animated way. What you say doesn't have to be especially clever or interesting – just keep up a running commentary of whatever it is you're both doing or seeing. Don't gabble non-stop, though. Stop, listen to her, and respond, making eye contact while you do so. The idea is to teach her that talking and communicating is a pleasurable thing. Gestures and actions – waving when you say 'goodbye' for instance – can help reinforce understanding. And reading, singing and reciting rhymes together are also great ways to help with language skills, especially if you repeat the same favourites regularly. Picture 'flashcards' are a great help, and can be fun, too.

Bear in mind that excessive dummy use can interfere with the development of babbling and talking, so it's best to make sure you limit it to night times and nap times at this stage. I'd also caution against too much television time for little ones who are just beginning to learn about language. Although limited viewing is fine and watching appropriate programmes or DVDs repeatedly can actually be useful in terms of learning, don't assume that hours in front of the goggle box will enhance your baby's communication skills! It's far better if she learns in real-life, and from you. (For more on television, see Question 48.)

What the netmums say

Baby talk

My son's first recognisable word was 'mumma'. He is nearly a year now and also says 'dadda', 'nanna', 'ganga' (grandad), and 'googir' (for good girl, said to any dog he sees!). When he's not using words we recognise, he babbles constantly, so he's obviously got a lot to say. We talk to him lots, and give him the opportunity to answer us, and we read to him loads, too. I'm an awful singer, but bless him, he loves my renditions of 'Row Your Boat', and 'Hickory Dickory Dock', and now tries to sing along with me. I love listening to him trying to talk.
Katrina from Hornchurch, mum to Isaac, eleven months

Joel was 'by the book' in his development. He did everything when they said he would, so I didn't have any worries until he was over a year old and not talking. After a year of stress and worry, he started talking at almost two – and then never stopped! By the time my little girl came along, I understood that babies developed at different rates, and never gave it a second thought. I have to say though that it was other people, not health visitors, who bugged me about it. Some people seemed to think his delay in talking was because he was stupid. One woman even suggested he was autistic. Erm, no, he is normal. Grrr!
Amy from Tyne and Wear, mum to Joel, three, and Charlotte, eighteen months

At eight and a half months, my daughter's first word was 'clap' – she said it as she was clapping, so there wasn't much doubt about it. I talk to her all the time as I think it's the best way to teach children about communication. She talks all the time too now. And I think it counts as a word if both you and your baby know what she's saying!
Ellen from Bath, mum to Lydia, twenty-one months

My oldest boy could only say two words by the time he was two: 'car' and 'ball'. I knew he was behind his peers, but didn't worry

too much as his understanding was fine. Then, at a routine check when he was two and half, the health visitor mentioned it. He was referred for speech therapy, but by the time the appointment for group sessions came through, about six months later, his speech had improved so much he didn't need them. My youngest says lots of words and is starting to string them together. I see now how behind my oldest was at the time, but I think I did the right thing by not worrying too much. He caught up in the end!
Jenny from Coventry, mum to James, four, and Alex, twenty-two months

Martha said her first words at eleven months. I say 'words', because she covered book, ball and balloon with a similar noise – we knew what she meant depending on the context! I had taken her to baby signing from five months, and I'm sure this contributed to her early speech. She was covering about twenty-five signs by the time she was talking – and I also found the signing great when she was talking but I couldn't understand what she was saying, as she would often sign and speak simultaneously. By fifteen months, she was saying about fifty words, and now, at three, she never stops. She even knows all the words to Abba songs!
Julia from Harrow, mum to Martha, three, and Tess, six months

Having said 'mum' and 'dad' quite early, my son said nothing else for a while, but at eighteen months, his speech is really starting to develop well. He particularly likes the word 'catch', when accompanied by the throwing of either a ball or himself! 'Nana' and 'banana' are also popular lately, as is 'bottle' and 'juice'. I've never been overly worried about his speech as I believe all children develop at their own pace, and I try not to judge his progress by the progress of others.
Clare from Doncaster, mum to Connor, eighteen months

I've always 'chatted back' to my little boy, initially with baby talk, but now he's older and starting to say words, I make sure I speak properly, like an adult should, so that he can hear how it's done. Even if I don't understand him when he talks – he can't say sentences yet, just odd words – I reply back with a sentence. I sing to him, too,

which he loves, although I am not the best singer in the world! I know that talking and interacting with him has helped him and he doesn't care whether I can hold a tune or not, or whether I understand him: he's just happy that I'm there, and interacting with him.
Di from Liverpool, mum to John, seventeen months

Eve had delayed speech. She was tested for autism, and received some speech therapy. As it turned out, she wasn't autistic and her speech came on in leaps and bounds when she started nursery. Charlie's speech developed normally, although occasionally now, he'll say something which we can't understand – like 'nookit', which turned out to be 'music'! At seven months, my youngest has just started babbling. She says 'mam-mam-mam', which is lovely!
Julie from Lichfield, mum to Eve, twelve, Charlie, two, and Amy, seven months

I was concerned about my son's speech to start with. He didn't talk till he was eighteen months old, and then said two words at once – 'dada' and 'dog'. He then learnt two words a month for three months, and by the time he was two he could say over fifty words, recognise colours, and count to six. I stopped worrying after that. My daughter said her first word at nine months ('mamma') and picked up words really quickly. She's just turned two, and has a large vocabulary. She sings along to nursery rhymes too, which is really sweet.
Natasha from Plymouth, mum to Kieran, four, and Livvy, two

My twins made all the usual 'Ma-ma, Da-da, Ba-ba,' noises first, at about six or seven months old. They used to babble to one another, which was sweet, and even now they have a kind of invisible language between them. They didn't seem to have any problems picking up words after their first ones. My third daughter said 'Dada' first, but then, rather than saying 'Mama' next, it was, 'What's that?' And this was by seven months old! She picked up language easily and was holding an understandable conversation at the age of thirteen months. At five, she still amazes me with her language.
Aimee from Chester, mum to Lauren and Megan, six, and Sophie, five

I was worried about my eldest. At his two-year check, he barely said a word. His vocabulary amounted to about ten words. Then he started nursery – and now I can't shut him up!

Karen from Warrington, mum to Matthew, two, and Katie, ten months

My daughter was very chatty even as a baby, always cooing and babbling or making a noise. She had well over 100 words by the time she was twenty months old and could make simple sentences from eighteen months. I like to think it's down to the time I spent reading and talking to her, but I think she is just one of life's talkative ones. She even mumbles in her sleep!

Alison from Weybridge, mum to Amelia, five

45 Why has he got so fussy about food?

If your little one took to weaning like a duck to water, and went on to chomp his way through a fantastic range of different tastes and textures with little persuasion, it's vexing if he starts refusing food. But fussy eating to one extent or another is extremely common in toddlers. There are various theories as to why, including one that they've been hotwired by evolution to start avoiding certain foods in case they're harmful. But most experts will tell you that food refusal is generally either a child's way of testing boundaries, of indulging their growing sense of independence or sometimes, frankly, a way to exert control over worried parents, in a world where they have precious little control over anything else. Of course, your little one could simply be developing different tastes, and learning about choice and preferences. And maybe he simply likes some things to eat, but not others – just like most adults.

Attitude is everything when it comes to living with a fussy eater, and your best bet is to stay calm and resilient in the face of fads. Thankfully, it's a situation that, for most, will improve over time. Meanwhile, bear in mind that it's normal, and it's common. If your little one has begun to turn his nose up at what's on his plate, and you are scraping your lovingly prepared offerings in the bin for the umpteenth time, take comfort in the thought that many other mums will be doing so, too.

What the experts say

Louise says: It can be really worrying if you've got a fussy eater and you're worried that he's not getting all his nutritional needs, but the truth is, he'll almost certainly survive this phase without any undue consequences for his health. I think it's a good idea to do a bit of research, and find out about the food groups and what makes a balanced diet, so that you can try to make sure he's getting at least something of everything. But really, you need to fight your anxiety on this, as it's likely to make the situation worse if your little one realises how much it matters to you. And the more you battle the more resistant he's likely to become.

Keep on serving up healthy options and be resilient about trying new things. With each meal, aim to give him something he will eat with something he might not. Sometimes you have to just give him what you know he will eat if you don't want him to starve, and that's fine. It might help to always make sure he's hungry when he comes to the table, so avoid letting him snack too close to meals. And if he's still having more than one or two milk feeds throughout the day, look to cut back on that as too much milk can suppress the appetite. It's worth bearing in mind, though, that toddlers' appetites can be erratic – they're often 'grazers', and may eat lots one day and little the next. They can also be satisfied with surprisingly small portions, and put off by large ones, so don't fill his plate up too full: you can always offer extra if he wants it. It's also worth taking a broader look at the diet you fear is really restrictive – it may be that, over the course of a week or two, he's getting a wider range of foods than you realise. Keep a food diary for a while and it could provide the reassurance you need.

Try stepping back and looking at the whole picture if you're worried about your fussy little eater's health. If he's developing and growing normally for his age, if he has energy, seems happy and isn't plagued with colds and minor infections, then there's unlikely to be anything wrong. By all means pop along to your GP for reassurance if you're really worried that some major nutritional needs are not being met. However, it's a rare case indeed when a doctor recommends specialist help for a toddler with fussy eating issues.

My own daughter went through this. Having been a great eater during weaning, she entered a very stressful phase of refusing everything, which left me feeling guilty, wondering what I'd done wrong, and frankly embarrassed to go to other homes where the children ate well! I even took to giving her a daily multivitamin supplement for a while, as I was so worried. She's better now, particularly when at nursery where there are other children to encourage her. I'm sure there'll be further improvements as she gets older but meanwhile, I've vowed not to get stressed out about it and we aim to eat as a family every day and make mealtimes as enjoyable as possible.

Crissy says: When your child refuses to eat your carefully prepared meal it can feel like a rejection not just of the food, but of you also. Fussy eating can cause a lot of worry and guilt for mums who fear they may be failing their child and then end up blaming themselves and their parenting skills for their toddler's pickiness. In truth, fussy eating and acting up at mealtimes is just as likely to be evidence of your child's hunger for independence as his disinterest in food. There aren't many areas of your toddler's life that he can claim to exert control over you, but food is one of them. As a parent, your responsibility is to provide your child with a varied and healthy diet, but you can't make him eat the food you put in front of him and if you try you're likely to do more harm than good, so give yourself a break.

Toddlers will generally eat when they're hungry and will often compensate for a skimpy meal at the next sitting, so they're very unlikely to starve themselves. Look at the bigger picture and consider what he's eaten over the course of a week rather than stressing over each individual mealtime and chances are you'll see that he's actually got a pretty balanced diet. It's very common for children of this age to stick to a few favourite foods while stubbornly rejecting others and toddlers are nothing if not inconsistent, so you'll often find that what's a hot favourite this week will be on his hate list the next.

If he prefers to play it safe on the food front don't try and force your little one to try new tastes. The average child will need to be repeatedly exposed to new foods before they become familiar enough to feel safe to sample them, so continue to offer new or previously rejected foods alongside his favourites, and let him know that he can choose to try them if and when he wants to.

Refusing food doesn't necessarily mean he hates it and will never come around to the idea, it usually just means he's still rather suspicious of it. He may not have the vocabulary to explain what it is that bothers him about a particular food and so it may simply be that he prefers his carrots crunchy and raw rather than cooked, or his pasta sauce puréed rather than lumpy, so don't give up at the first hurdle. Try presenting the same food in a different guise. Some children seem to have particularly sensitive taste buds and won't like stronger tasting or smelling foods, while others will take against a food just because they don't like the texture or the colour, or because it reminds them of the time when they had chicken pox or the dog barked and scared them. If your child sees that you're taking his food refusal in your stride he's more likely to lose interest in the whole business, so if he says he's not hungry, he's full or he doesn't like what's on offer don't offer him an alternative or let him fill up on snacks, just grit your teeth and clear the table.

Supporting your child to learn to eat well is about more than nutrition; it's also about helping him develop a healthy emotional relationship with food. So avoid presenting food in terms of punishment or reward and don't withhold it when he's behaving badly or use pudding or sweets to bribe your toddler into eating his veg. It's also worth taking a good hard look at the example you're setting your child. If you're continually snacking on junk food, talking about your next diet or you're a grazer who never sits still long enough for a proper meal, how can you seriously expect your toddler to opt for healthy foods, finish his dinner or sit nicely to the table? Wherever possible, take the time to sit down and eat with your toddler, minimise distractions by banning toys and television at the table, and involve him in making choices, shopping and food preparation. I'm not suggesting you make food faces or sculptures out of mashed potato, which is a lot of hard work, but try to make food fun whenever possible. Adopt a leisurely pace at mealtimes and don't rush him, hover or start clearing away while he's still eating, so your toddler gets the message that mealtimes are not a trial or a chore, but an opportunity for sociable family time. Let him experiment with his food – even if he ends up mashing banana in his hair. You can always pop him in the bath later!

What the netmums say

Food fights

My daughter used to eat everything. And then, at two, I don't know what went wrong, but she started to refuse food. Even now she'll only eat from a select number of meals, and is not willing to try anything new. I hide veg in her meals though and thankfully, she's always liked fruit. So far, my son will try anything. I am yet to find something he *won't* eat!
Megan from Edinburgh, mum to Carly, four, and Stuart, fourteen months

After weaning, my daughter ate well and enjoyed a wide variety of flavours – in fact, it was often the stronger flavours that she preferred, and she still loves ginger in all its forms. But as I started to bring in more texture, she would gag and sometimes just bring back the whole lot. I would now class her as fussy. There are certain meals she will eat (although often only with a measure of coercion), but she's a nightmare for trying anything new. We tell her she has to give it a lick, at the very least, which she'll do pretty readily but will usually then refuse to have more. We don't give her alternative meals, and she doesn't really snack in between. Some weeks she'll eat well, and the next she doesn't want to know, but I suppose over a month she does OK. She's a healthy weight, has plenty of energy, is generally very happy, sleeps the night through, and is rarely ill, so I think she must be getting all she needs right now.
Helen from Bexleyheath, mum to Amber, two

My middle child was fine until he got to ten months old, when he started refusing foods. Gradually his list of liked foods got shorter, and by eleven months we were on to a fairly limited, fixed menu. Every breakfast had to be porridge, and so did most lunches (although he might have fruit purée in it). His range of dinners was small – all dairy- and carb-based. By the time he was one, there were few foods he liked. We have a picture of him with his first birthday cake, but he wouldn't eat dessert by then (except

yoghurts), and once he'd blown out the candles he refused to eat any! There was no particular trigger for this fussiness. And he's still extremely fussy now, at five. We've tried just about everything, including making everything into a curry (which worked for a while); gradually expanding his menu bit by bit; blending disliked foods into foods he did eat (which didn't work – in fact, when he detected puréed veg in mince he just stopped eating mince); always putting a small amount of disliked food on his plate and ignoring whether he ate it or not (that didn't work – he just refused to eat anything until all traces of the offending food were gone from his plate); and refusing to dish up anything special for him (he then didn't eat for four days and by then he was sleepy; it scared me, and I caved in). He's fussy about a lot of things besides food, and his dad is too, so I think it's just down to his personality.
Abi from Mitcham, mum to Alice, eight, Byron, five, and Phoenix, eight months

When my daughter suddenly started turning things down – particularly veg – we overcame it by sprinkling 'fairy dust' on her plate, i.e. edible glitter, made for cake decorating. I told her the magic will only work if she eats all her veggies and it seemed to do the trick. Now she'll even ask to try new ones. If she's not keen, I try again in a few weeks.
Charlotte from Ellesmere, mum to Evelyn, three

Kip was always fussy. After weaning him at six months, he refused to eat a proper meal until he was about nine months old – he'd developed an incredibly strong tongue thrust, so anything that went in came straight back out. The next stage was finding food that smelled good – Kip was a 'sniffer', and still is. And woe betide me if the food was the wrong colour. Or texture. Or shape. Or temperature. We scrapped like mad for a few years, and I got it all wrong – gave in, lost my temper, bribed him. But now I've got too many other things to worry about and I've decided to choose my battles. He loves fruit, so he can have as much of that as he likes. We eat together when we can, with choices where possible, and I have a laissez-faire approach to 'treats'. He's as lean and as strong as they come, his skin, hair and teeth are healthy, and he's growing. My advice is, always have a bottle of tomato sauce to hand, and a bag of chocolate buttons in your pocket.

Hannah from Whitley Bay, mum to Ted, seven, Kip, five, and Annis, two

Both my children have been through fussy phases, usually about the same time as they show other behaviours that appear to be control- and independence-related, such as tantrums. I dealt with it by continuing to offer a wide range of foods, ensuring that there was always something on their plate that they did like, but never going out of my way not to serve foods they wouldn't eat. They would then have the choice to eat it or not eat it, and if they didn't, I would not get upset – or at least, let them see me get upset, by their refusal to eat. Regardless of whether they eat or not, they have to stay at the table until everyone else has finished. More often than not they get bored and end up finishing what's on their plate anyway.

Stacey from Chester, mum to Heather, three, and Lorelai, seventeen months

As babies, mine both ate everything. My son didn't care what was going in his mouth; he would eat whole bowls of homemade stuff, no matter what it was. My daughter was also a good little eater. Fussiness started with both of them around ten months, when they started to develop some language skills. However, although they were weaned on the same foods, my son wants to eat nothing but toast and toast-like stuff, while my daughter only wants to eat veg. The end result is that they can share a meal – Albie will eat all the unhealthy stuff and Evie will eat the rest! We always eat as a family and I will only make one meal. It's a take-it-or-leave-it approach; if they don't want to eat, then that's fine. I sometimes try to encourage them to try something they would not usually touch, but promising more of the food they love. Albie quite often goes along with that. If he does not eat any of his meal, he never ever gets a pudding. We do not force them to eat anything, but they do go without now and again.

Marion from Macclesfield, mum to Albie, two, and Evie, fifteen months

My daughter would eat anything I gave her at the weaning stage. However, as she's become more able to indicate choice and express likes and dislikes, the list of things she doesn't like has got longer and longer. It also changes on a weekly basis! She tends to go through 'fads' where she'll eat the same thing every day for weeks and then overnight will decide she doesn't like it. I myself was an extremely fussy eater as a child. My overriding memory is being forced by a school dinner lady to eat platefuls of cold veg, and I want to make sure my daughter never sees mealtimes as a battle or food as the enemy (or a comfort), and in an age where eating disorders are prevalent I do not want her relationship with food to be fraught from the start. So if my daughter decides she doesn't like anything then it's no biggie, as long as she eats something. I don't care if it's pasta for tea thirty days in a row! I feel that the bigger a deal you make of it, the bigger a deal it becomes. I'm sure it will pan out as she gets older, especially at school when she sees what other kids eat and she can be more logical about it. She's healthy and has hit all her milestones, and she certainly has plenty of energy. Unless it becomes a medical or developmental issue, then I will stick with this attitude.

Amanda from Runcorn, mum to Emily, three

We encountered issues thanks to my son's violent reflux. He became frightened of certain foods if he believed he would be sick because of eating them. We made a point of only ever offering healthy options, so he couldn't get addicted to sugary or fast foods. We also persisted with offering the foods he was scared of, and eventually he would try a small amount of them. Other times he ignored it and ate whatever else was on his plate. I really do believe persistence does pay off and that there's no need to cave in to their demands for favourite foods. If they're hungry they will eat what's on their plate.

Hayley from Staines, mum to Jay, four

My daughter used to eat almost anything but in the past nine months has become fussy. Recently we've had a bit of success by saying, 'I bet you can't eat your sausage,' then, when she does eat it, we look surprised and give her lots of praise. She finds this hilarious and so she eats even more to provoke a similar reaction. My only concern is that in time if we overuse this method, she may start to think we have no faith in her ability to do things. For now, it just seems to be a good way to get some food down her!

Helen from Carlisle, mum to Louise, two, and Joseph, two months

46 How can we get shot of the dummy?

Accepted wisdom is that it's best to help your baby drop her dummy habit altogether before the age of one, mainly because too much dummy-sucking will reduce her opportunities to babble, and to practise all the mouth movements and speech sounds she needs to develop her talking skills. There's also the argument that the sooner you take it away, the easier it will be to do so. And if you're frequently required to get up in the night to help her locate her dummy when she loses it, perhaps that's motivation enough to get shot of it.

Some parents are happy to let their babies keep their dummies well into the toddling years, and that's OK if the habit is carefully moderated. If your baby just sucks her dummy at night and at nap-time, for example, and perhaps occasionally in the day when she's looking for a cuddle and some comfort, then it's not going to cause any long-term problems. And it has to be said that one advantage in waiting until they're a bit older is that you can enlist the services of the 'dummy fairy', or ask Father Christmas to take her dummy away for the Lapland babies, in exchange for a Christmas present. When it comes down to it, a lot of parents are pleasantly surprised by how well their little ones cope when their dummy is taken away. But do always pick your time carefully. Don't take away a source of comfort at a time when she's poorly, teething, or going through a phase of separation anxiety or other upheaval such as you returning to work or a house move.

What the experts say

Louise says: Speech and language therapists have serious concerns that too much dummy sucking can affect language development, and – if the habit is very frequent, and prolonged – dentists warn that it could have an effect on the alignment of the teeth. You only have to worry about these risks if your baby does a lot of dummy-sucking, but even so, I advise aiming to cut pacifier use out altogether before she's one, and in the meantime, to make sure use is well restricted. Don't put a dummy in your baby's mouth unless she actually needs it for comfort or to get herself off to sleep!

When it comes to ditching the dummy, you may want to take a gradual approach – particularly if your baby relies on hers a lot and you don't think you can bear the fallout if you just take it away abruptly. However, to my mind, the best solution is to go 'cold turkey', in other words, removing the dummy altogether and dealing with the consequences as best you can. It can make for a difficult few days, and you'll probably need to be prepared to offer alternative forms of comfort and distraction, such as extra cuddles and play. Taking a dummy away at night-time can be trickier still and if your baby needs to suck hers to get her off to sleep you may, if she's old enough, have to use some gentle sleep training techniques to wean her off this sleep association (see Question 35).

Having said all that, I don't have a problem with babies holding on to their dummies into the toddling years, as long as it's a habit that is carefully restricted. Ideally, once past one, you'd only be offering your little one her dummy at night-time and perhaps for naps too. And some parents feel it's easier to take a dummy away from an older child, because at least you can use reasoning then, or perhaps a tried and tested psychological ploy like the recruitment of the 'dummy fairy'. If you go down this route, be open about what you're doing, and chat about how grown-up children don't need dummies, which is an approach that usually appeals. You might even find if you wait a while that you don't need to take steps to remove a dummy at all, as lots of little ones will get to the point where they ditch it for themselves anyway.

If your baby's long-term comfort habit is thumb-sucking, there may be more serious implications for her teeth, as thumb-sucking can sometimes carry on for years, potentially pushing the adult teeth out of alignment. Still, there's not too much to be done about thumb-sucking, as unlike a dummy, you can't very well take a thumb away. Try not to fret, or nag her to stop, as that may just have the opposite effect. In most cases, a child will drop this habit of her own accord, eventually. Meanwhile, if you're really concerned, try offering distraction whenever you can.

As for other comforters like blankets or much-loved soft toys, I would say don't worry about it if your baby's attachment to hers stays with her well into toddlerhood. It's probably a good idea to gently discourage it at times other than when she's comfort-seeking though, in case it's hampering her chances of playing or learning – and because you probably won't want her taking it to school with her when the time comes!

What the netmums say

Ditching the dummy

My daughter loved her dummies and counted each one before bed. She would wake and cry until all six were found – and once, she screamed for an hour on a plane when she lost just one of them. So I was dreading taking them away. The dentist suggested we get rid of them, when she was two. We mentioned it a few times in front of her, and then one day just went for it, waiting for the tears and tantrums, but nothing. There were a few tears at bedtime, but I think our assertive approach worked. In return she got a new toy. With my son, we never felt we needed a dummy. He gets comfort from rubbing my arm and snuggling my neck!
Melanie from Retford, mum to Satya, four, and Joshua, two

Amelie had her dummy until she was nearly two. As she got older, she only had it to settle to sleep and most of the time would throw it out of bed! As they started to wear out, we decided to get rid of them. She called them 'num nums' and so one weekend we took her to Bear Factory and let her choose a toy, which we named

Num Num, to replace those that we were getting rid of. When she went to bed she could take Num Num puppy with her instead of the dummies and we had no trouble at all.
Teresa from Paddock Wood, mum to Amelie, four, and Juliette, seven months

I took his dummy away for the first time at seven months. We just stopped it, cold turkey, which worked for a month, but then we relapsed as he was waking for teething and we couldn't cope with the lack of sleep, so gave it back. Stupid, really. At nine months we did it properly – cold turkey again, which caused a bit of crying in the night but I'm not sure he really missed it. I don't regret giving it to him, though. I think he used it to satisfy his sucking reflex and got it out of his system, so he's never gone for his thumb.
Christine from York, mum to Matthew, eleven months

At two, we told our son that the hospital had lots of new babies who didn't have dummies, so they were sad and crying, and that if Owen posted his dummies to them, they would be really happy. To our amazement, he gladly put all of them into a large envelope and posted them through our front door. He did ask us for the next couple of nights where they were, but we kept reminding him of the story. He was so proud that he'd helped the babies.
Emma from Okehampton, mum to Owen, three

I restricted the use of a dummy just to bedtime at eighteen months, and then when Josh was three years old we put it under the Christmas tree for Santa so he could give it to other little boys and girls. Santa then kindly left him some presents, as a thank you! It worked really well.
Calley from Haywards Heath, mum to Josh, eight, and Jack, two

Callum had started to bite through the teat, so one afternoon I cut the teat of his last dummy and left it on the coffee table. He found the dummy on the table, and said that it was broken, so I said that it would have to go in the bin. He agreed, put the dummy in the bin himself, and has never had a dummy since.
Leanne from Stevenage, mum to Callum, four

We used that magic ingredient, fairy dust, to rid our daughter of her dummy at eighteen months old. After sprinkling glitter in the garden so they knew where to go, we put all the dummies into the magic bag and went out. When we got back, the dummies had gone and she had a baby fairy doll waiting for her. She asked for it once after, but changed her mind when we said we would have to send the fairy back!

Charlotte from Ellesmere, mum to Evelyn, three

My son loved his dummy, and I'm such a softy, I just let him have it for as long as he wanted. Just after his fourth birthday he bit it and broke it, so I told him we had to throw it away, which he did. And that was it – no more dummy! I let him give up in his own time, and I think he would have been so upset doing it before he was ready. There was no rush.

Tracy from London, mum to Jamel, four

Kieran still had his dummy at bedtime at two. We were going to a theme park for the day, and knew Peppa Pig and George Pig were going to be there. So we got all his dummies and explained to him that because George was a baby and Kieran was a big boy, George needed dummies more than Kieran did so we should leave them there for him. He asked a couple of times at bedtime for his dummy, but other than that, dummies were never mentioned again!

Nicola from Swindon, mum to Kieran, three

I decided to go with my mum's tried-and-tested strategy – taking away the dummy after the first birthday party, and going cold turkey! I started talking about it when they were ten months, not knowing whether or not they understood what I was saying. Their actual birthday was a weekday and we had the party on the Saturday. They both had their dummies in the morning and forgot about them once the party started. When it was time to go to bed, they slept fine without then, and I threw them away that evening. I was tempted to keep two in case it all got a bit too much the next day, but they didn't seem to mind at all.

Nkaepe from Leeds, mum to Ebun and Ore, two

47 When will he stop napping?

Most babies continue to need a certain amount of daytime napping to make up their full quota of needed sleep well into toddlerhood. Typically, they drop from two or three naps a day to one single (but substantial) chunk of daytime sleep some time after their first birthday, and drop napping altogether by the age of three. But you may well find your little one needs more or less daytime sleep than is average, and drops his napping entirely either sooner or later than the norm.

Nap-time can be a huge boon for parents, allowing a little time to get stuff done, devote themselves to siblings, or simply have a cuppa and a re-charge. On the other hand, it can be a nuisance having to make time for naps when you've got lots of other stuff you need to do (although with a pushchair, you can often meet both demands at the same time). Truth is, by this stage naps are something your little one will either take or won't, and there's not a great deal you can do to influence it either way. If your baby's still napping, it's probably because he still needs to, and if he's stopped napping, he probably doesn't need them any more. Try to go with the flow on this one, and let your baby lead the way.

What the experts say

Maggie says: As time goes on, the amount of sleep your baby needs per twenty-four hours will reduce gradually, which means his daytime napping will decrease. It's very variable, though – some babies seem to function normally without much in the way of daytime sleep, and give up on napping well before their second birthday. Others need to nap for longer, or more frequently, and will still be happily indulging in a good nap aged three or four. He might only stop because his day is too full of other things to allow for some shut-eye!

When it comes to daytime napping, it's best to let your baby lead the way as far as your lives will allow – and of course, lives tend to get busier the older babies get, so it can sometimes be hard or even impossible to fit nap-time in, not least because daycare arrangements don't always allow for it. However, as a general rule, if your little one's still napping in the day, it's because he needs to, so if you can facilitate it, then do. After lunch is a good natural point to encourage napping as you have nature on your side – it's now that the body clock winds down. There's a good reason why many Europeans take a 'siesta' in the early afternoon!

Your little one will drop his naps altogether when he no longer requires them, and it will become obvious when he's ready to do so: you'll put him in his cot and he'll object, or will simply sit there playing and singing to himself rather than lying down and dropping off! For a while, you may well notice a pattern when your baby refuses to sleep for several days, but will then have a 'catch-up'. Some babies will also start to 'fight' being put down for naps, even though technically they're tired and really need one. It's not unusual; it just means he's at a point where he knows there are more interesting options available. In these cases, there's not much point in forcing it. You might find yourself resorting to a walk or drive, if you know he'll drop off in the pushchair or in his car seat. But if that's not possible, you'll probably just have to steel yourself for a tough time a bit later on when he becomes cranky – and you may need to call on all your powers of distraction to get him through the final period before bedtime.

You might wonder if purposefully cutting out or cutting down your baby's daytime naps will help you get more sleep at night, or an earlier bedtime for him, or more of a lie-in in the mornings. But I'd always advise against forcing your baby to stay awake when he needs sleep. If he's slumbering on until late in the afternoon, and you know you're likely to struggle to get him down at bedtime as a result, then it's probably a good idea to cut his nap short. But generally speaking, babies are pretty good at moderating their own sleep needs. And in fact, getting the amount of nap-time he needs in the day will usually help your baby sleep well at night, not the other way round, since he's more likely to settle well at bedtime and sleep soundly through the night if he's *not* overtired.

What the netmums say

Dropping naps

My little boy naps for two hours in the morning. He's only just dropped his afternoon nap but gets really tired around 6 p.m., so bath-time has had to be moved to mornings as he's just too tired to cope with it in the evening.
Christine from Bolton, mum to Jack, fourteen months

Violet dropped down to one lunchtime nap at around a year old and then stopped napping altogether just after her second birthday. I'd put her in her cot and instead of going to sleep she'd just play and chat for an hour or so! She did then sleep for thirteen to fourteen hours at night, so it wasn't all bad.
Catherine from Nottingham, mum to Violet, two

Carly always slept for an hour in the morning and an hour in the afternoon, before dropping all naps at three years old. My son dropped down from three to two naps when he was five months old and now he has one nap at about 12.30 p.m., usually an hour, sometimes longer, depending on what time he's up in the morning. I think nap-time continues to be important if your child is up early. He certainly gets very grumbly when he's tired, so I always know when he needs a nap. It also gives me time to spend alone with my daughter.
Megan from Edinburgh, mum to Carly, four, and Stuart, fourteen months

Matthew is still having two naps a day – about an hour in the morning and an hour in the afternoon. I used to have to rock him to get him to nap, and then he would only take really short naps several times

a day. But once he started crawling I just started putting him in his cot – and miraculously he started having these regular naps!
Christine from York, mum to Matthew, eleven months

My little girl has only had one nap during the day since she was about eight months old. She'll only sleep for half an hour to fifty minutes maximum in the day now, and usually that will be in her pushchair.
Darla from Solihull, mum to Lola, nineteen months

Most days now, Cian has one nap. Sometimes if he's really sleepy he'll have two, and some days, he'll not sleep at all. But he always goes to his bed at 7.30 p.m. every night and sleeps till 8 a.m., so I don't mind so much if he's not slept during the day.
Vicki from Glasgow, mum to Cian, fourteen months

As a young baby, Kieran would only sleep for twenty minutes at a time during the day and I had no time to myself to get things done. He would *only* sleep in his crib at home, and I had to rock him to sleep. I can't remember when he dropped his late afternoon sleep, but he went down to one lunchtime sleep at twelve months, and for that he slept for two hours. Finally I could get some house-work done or sit down and relax, which was great! He dropped this sleep altogether at two and a half years. My daughter on the other hand slept all the time as a baby, and would also fall asleep anywhere. She also went down to one lunchtime sleep at twelve months old, and also slept for two hours. She still does. I enjoy this break as she is always on the go and it's the only chance I get to sit down during the day.
Natasha from Plymouth, mum to Kieran, four, and Livvy, two

My first two dropped their morning naps by about twenty months, and kept their afternoon nap until the age of about two and a half. My third dropped her morning naps by about eight months, and dropped both by the time she was one. She was just too nosey, and obviously thought she was going to miss something! Daytime naps have always been a godsend for me. Just getting to drink a hot cup of tea or even just sitting for five minutes was heaven. It was a great time to recharge myself ready for the next lot of feeding/changing/playing. Mine were all pretty good daytime sleepers: I just placed them in their beds, and they went off to sleep. And if we were out and about, they'd sleep in the car or the buggy.

Aimee from Chester, mum to Lauren and Megan, six, and Sophie, five

My twins never had more than one nap in the day. One of them dropped hers at eighteen months, which I found hard as it was my only chance to get anything done. The other would probably still have one if I let her, and they're four now.

Jo from Banbury, mum to Olivia and Lily, four

It's starting to get very difficult to put Ryan down for a nap now – he really fights it, although when it does get to afternoon time and he hasn't had a sleep, we can all tell, as he's so grumpy and unreasonable.

Alyssa from Leeds, mum to Ryan, twenty months

Joseph tends to take himself off to bed for a nap just after lunch-time. I wake him after an hour or so because he will sleep for two or three hours if allowed and then he's less likely to sleep at night. He definitely needs some kip in the day, though, as he's a very active boy and he gets very grumpy when tired.

Kelly from Lymm, mum to Joseph, twenty-one months

My son still naps for an hour and a half to two hours in the after-noon. It doesn't seem to affect his night-time sleep – he goes to bed at eight and sleeps until eight the next the morning. He's like me; he likes his sleep.

Kayleigh from London, mum to Ryan, two

48 Is it OK to let her watch telly?

It's a rare toddler who hasn't discovered the joys of TV viewing – and a rare parent who hasn't realised that turning it on will almost always offer a short period of time in which to take a breather, or to get something necessary done. But is it bad for them? Some experts do express concern about telly time for toddlers, mainly based on fears that too much could hinder developing speech and language skills – and, in the case of seriously bad television habits, at the expense of their taking part in other activities, too. A few have even spoken out to recommend that parents of pre-schoolers keep it off the menu altogether. Meanwhile, back in the real world, how are you supposed to explain away the grey box in the corner (and, no doubt, your own viewing habits)? Fortunately for busy parents, most sensible people seem to agree that telly for toddlers is absolutely fine in small, carefully monitored doses. And after all, there are also positives to television: it can be educational, as well as entertaining.

There aren't any firm or official guidelines when it comes to your toddler watching television, although the National Literacy Trust suggests a limit of no more than half an hour of 'appropriate' daily viewing for tots under two. Ultimately, it's down to you to decide what to let your little one tune in to, and when.

What the experts say

Louise says: There's no doubt that TV can be a useful thing when you need to get something done, or just to grab a breather. My advice with toddlers is to try and limit it to short spurts, say half an hour at a time, no more than once or twice a day. You definitely don't want it on all day because that's going to restrict the wide range of different play and activities she needs for healthy development. And in particular, some speech and language experts believe it's not a good way for little ones to learn language, which is far better acquired via two-way communication, with an interested adult. There is thought to be benefit, though, in repetitive watching of the same DVD or programme, so if your little one likes to replay the same viewing material over and over, that's probably a good thing. My own daughter was obsessed with *Mary Poppins* for a while, and learned much of the dialogue and songs by heart!

Other useful guidelines are not to have the television on during mealtimes – it's healthier all round to sit at the table as a family and to relax and chat over your food – and not to let kids of any age have televisions in the bedroom. I'd also advise strongly against having the TV on in the background. Switch it off in between viewings, even if your child is occupied with some other activity. She's very likely to be distracted by it and it's better if she can focus completely on what she's doing, whether that's drawing, role-play, building bricks, or having a conversation with you. It's also a good idea to turn off televisions in the run-up to bedtime as they can cause over-stimulation, which could affect sleep.

Make sure what your toddler is exposed to is appropriate; in other words, programmes and films made specifically for young children. There's some great stuff on the television schedules for young children these days, so pick carefully. Choose good-quality programmes from channels like CBeebies, and you won't go far wrong. Make sure you know at all times what she's watching – sticking with pre-recorded stuff and DVDs is a good way to vet her viewing.

Crissy says: For a busy mum juggling childcare, work and household chores it requires an iron will to resist using television as a babysitter in a box. Sitting your toddler down in front of CBeebies for a while can buy you a chance to draw breath – particularly if there's a new baby in the house. In recent years, however, compelling research-based evidence has emerged to suggest that excessive television viewing in the very early childhood years, a critical period for brain development, may be detrimental to our children's intellectual, linguistic and social development, and could even affect their long-term physical health, behaviour and sleep patterns. As a parent, you might wonder if it's OK to switch on at all.

In most families, it would be unrealistic to introduce a total ban on TV for toddlers. Fortunately there's plenty of quality programming available to your child that can be educational as well as entertaining and can introduce new ideas, skills and experiences. The problems come when too much viewing takes away from time that could be better spent on more beneficial and enriching play activities, so it's important to limit your little one's viewing time to short sessions and take care to balance sofa time with one-to-one active and interactive play. Setting clear boundaries for when it's OK to watch television can also be helpful. Banning television from the bedroom or during meals is one way you might try doing this. Try not to sit down and idly flick through the channels until something appeals; instead select a specific programme or DVD and in the interests of family harmony remember to signpost the end of TV time, always letting her know what you're going to do when the programme finishes. Too much exposure to fast-moving images can affect concentration skills, so look instead for age-appropriate, interactive programmes with a gentle pace that offer her the chance to join in with singing, dancing and story-telling, rather than sitting immobile staring at the screen.

No doubt there'll be times when in the interests of your own sanity your toddler will end up watching TV on her own for a while, but wherever possible, even if you have to resort to bringing your laptop or ironing board into the room, try to share viewing time and join in, so she gets the clear message that you care what she watches.

What the Netmums say

On the box

We don't have the TV on in the daytime, but Eleanor has a bunch of DVDs (for instance, The Wiggles) that are invaluable if she's too tired to amuse herself while we get dinner ready. When she was a bit younger we used them practically every day but now she's getting more absorbed in games, they don't go on so much. But the rule is, they go off as soon as she gets interested in something else. She's not really the square-eyed type – she'll often just crawl off and play in the middle of something, which is good!
Susannah from York, mum to Eleanor, fourteen months

My little boy watches telly. Sometimes we sit and watch it together and we talk about what's happening on the screen and sing along, and sometimes he likes to sit on his own on the couch and watch while I do the ironing, or simply have five minutes to myself. I don't really need to restrict it as he'll only watch it for a wee while, then come away himself to do other things. We go out at least once a day so he's never ever sitting in front of the telly all day. I think we've struck a pretty good balance.
Marianne from Uddingston, mum to William, twenty-two months

Bethany took an interest in TV from about six months. She took notice of *Something Special* and *In the Night Garden*, which has become part of her bedtime routine. I allow her some TV time in the morning after breakfast while she gets dressed, then she watches *Balamory* before lunch, has half an hour before tea, and *In The Night Garden* at bedtime. I'm careful not to keep it on all day and would not let her have a television in her bedroom, which doubles up as her playroom. I don't think her viewing has stunted her development as she enjoys books, talks well and is very engaged socially. She seems to have learnt some sign language too!
Ruth from Newton Abbot, mum to Bethany, seventeen months, and Thomas, five months

Lawrence has always watched TV, but only ever pre-recorded stuff from the digi-box, and usually only about half an hour a day. I pre-record, mainly because I can't stand adverts and also because I just find some children's programmes so awful.
Helen from the Isle of Wight, mum to Lawrence, two

The TV is always on in our house. Both boys can take or leave it and will alternate between watching whatever's on and playing with their toys. Damien surprised me the other day by counting to eight in Spanish, courtesy of *Handy Manny*. He's now teaching me! I think as soon as you start to restrict something they want it more and it becomes a big deal. I do monitor what they watch, though. Damien went through a phase of being really into *Ben 10* but I became concerned that it was making him aggressive, so we stopped it. They've learned things from television that I could never have taught them.
Yvonne from Ayr, mum to Damien, four, and Quinn, two

We don't have a TV licence, but we let our son watch up to an hour of a DVD in the evening as a wind-down before bed. I do think TV can become a 'lazy parenting tool' and didn't want to fall into that myself during the day, and I've read reports that suggest more than two hours of TV a day could be damaging. I want my son to learn to use his imagination, play creatively and also experience the innocence of childhood. And not having a licence means we can shelter him from things like the news, which I don't think is suitable for his age. However we never make an issue of TV or 'forbid' it, as then it would become very attractive. Rather, we will turn it off if his interest goes on to something else and offer options in the evening of a DVD or a book – he often chooses a book or ten minutes of watching and then a book. We've tried to encourage him to watch educational programmes on DVD, too, but *Finding Nemo* always wins! I think TV is a great thing to give new experiences, but only if used in moderation.
Rebecca from Ammanford, mum to Noah, two

My daughter tunes into the children's programmes a few times a day, and sometimes I can switch it off and she won't even notice because she's too busy doing something else. I think TV has its place in toddlers' development. I am constantly talking to her and teaching her, but the television has also taught her lots of words and helps her recognise all sorts of things – wild animals, for instance – that she would not see in everyday life. I monitor what's on if she's around when we've got the television on, because she is of a mind now to pay more attention to it and copy words that I don't want her to learn!

Anita from Swindon, mum to Freya, eighteen months

To be honest, it has really helped having CBeebies since the arrival of Anya's baby brother. Being a single parent can be tough and if you can grab half an hour to yourself thanks to *Mr Tumble* or *Charlie and Lola*, then I think it makes for a happier and peaceful household. Now that her brother is going a bit longer between feeds and the better weather is here we spend more time out and about but she still really enjoys watching her bit of telly to relax after a busy day at the park.

Claire from Spalding, mum to Anya, three, and Aidan, two months

I used to be very against small children watching TV, and my daughter didn't have any until she was two. She was a very active child, I took her out a lot, and she was always happy playing at home, so I didn't see the need. However, now I'm pregnant and feeling sick a lot so I've given in. Initially it was just a couple of shows a day (which I think is ideal) and she has some DVDs, but it's sometimes on for a few hours at a time. I still worry it's lazy parenting, but on the other hand I have no energy. It's a case of needs must!

Emma from Bournemouth, mum to Sophie, two

Both my children watch television, but we are also very active. We go out more or less every day, either to playgroup, soft play, or friends' homes, and they also both have activities. But when we come home, the television goes on. They usually watch the Disney channel, or Nick Jr. However, they're not stuck to it like zombies – although it's often on in the background, they will also be playing, messing around, drawing or just up to no good! They love their TV shows, and why shouldn't they? As long as it's not just an electric babysitter, I think it's OK. Sometimes we're extremely naughty and eat treats while we watch it, too!

Rachael from Bristol, mum to Olivia, three, and Theo, sixteen months

My daughter was fascinated by *Waybuloo* from as early as three months. She then went through a *Chuggington* phase and now seems to like a variety of programmes. I have a stock of them recorded on the Sky box ready for an emergency. I think she gets a lot out of it when she watches it in short snaps. I reckon it's good for her language development if I chat along with her about what's happening. She also enjoys dancing and singing along. I do limit it though, and would never have it on just in the background. I know for a fact that this affects her concentration – she will get totally distracted by the television and not join in with a conversation, or will stop playing. I don't like the way she seems mesmerised by it. She has about half an hour after breakfast, which allows me to get dressed and do the washing up, and she usually has another half an hour in the evening, before her bath.

Nicky from Camberley, mum to Ella, twenty-three months

49 When should I start toilet training?

When your little one becomes ready to leave his nappy days behind depends entirely on him. Learning to control the bowel and bladder requires a combination of physical, social and emotional readiness, which most children reach somewhere between two and three. Waiting until he's showing the right signs is key if you don't want to put him off the whole idea completely. And patience in this matter is very likely to pay: if you wait until he's completely confident, and mature enough to take this step in his stride, it's more likely to be a speedy, straightforward process when the time comes – with fewer accidents likely, too.

Arm yourself with a good sense of humour and a resigned outlook for toilet training. Before you've finished, there's very likely to be wee or poo in places where you didn't really want it. That's life.

What the experts say

Louise says: A good marker that your little one is ready for toilet training is if he seems agitated or uncomfortable in a nappy that's either wet or dirty. It's difficult to put an age range on when that might be, as there's such a variable timescale on this. A few will be ready from eighteen months onwards, but somewhere between two and three is more typical.

Aim to introduce him to the whole concept well in advance. Take him to the loo with you, let him have a little sit on it if he wants, and chat about it naturally, whenever he has done a pee or a poo. I seem to recall actually sitting on my daughter's potty myself when toilet training her, just to show her how it's done! Your best bet is to make it fun – lots of parents find that encouraging their little one to look at a book or sing a song whilst on the potty can help to make a positive experience of it. Never make him sit there endlessly if he's not happy or it's clear nothing's happening. And make sure he can give it a go at any time, should the urge take him – leave potties in several accessible places, and when he seems ready to use the loo itself, put a child-size seat on the toilet, and have a small footstool nearby that will help him reach it.

When the time comes, go out and buy lots of cheap pants, a couple of children's books on the subject, and several potties, if you don't have them already. It's up to you whether you go for an intensive technique, or a more relaxed and gradual approach over several months – but if he's ready, it can usually be cracked in a week or two, or even a weekend. Good weather's a bonus, as you can let him wander round nappy-less outside and not have to worry about mess too much. You'll soon work out what the signals are when he needs to go, if you don't know already. Look for wriggling, or the usual facial expressions, and gently remind him if necessary. It's also worth nudging him if you know it's a time when he would usually go. But try to avoid constantly asking if he needs the potty, though, as he could probably do without the irritation.

If it's just not happening, there's no shame in stopping, putting him back in nappies, and trying again a bit later. And don't worry about backtracking if you need to because he's regressed having had it sussed previously, which can easily happen when some emotional or practical upheaval upsets him. It happened to my previously dry daughter after we moved house, and I put her back in nappies and just tried again a few months later. Do bear that in mind when you're picking the right time to try toilet training – don't attempt it if you know there's anything round the corner.

Maggie says: It's a very individual thing, when a child is ready to be toilet trained, but for the majority it will come at age two plus. Unfortunately a lot of mums feel under artificial pressure to get their child toilet trained, perhaps so that they're dry for pre-school or because other children they know have got there already. But it's so important not to rush a little one into pants, because it can be counterproductive – usually when toilet training turns out to be protracted or difficult, it's because parents have tried it too early. Often parents are 'toilet timing' rather than toilet training, and it's a different thing. If you simply plonk him on the potty or loo when he's due for one, you probably will be lucky sometimes – and sometimes you won't! What you want is for him to be spontaneously managing and controlling the situation for himself, and he'll only be able to do that when his central nervous system is sufficiently matured. In other words, he needs to be able to recognise when his bladder is full, or that he needs a poo, and for that message to get to his brain in time to act. It's a complex business, and one that has nothing to do with intelligence!

So, my main advice is to wait until he's ready, and that will be when he's showing the right signs. Usually that's when he's conscious of being wet or dirty; that he understands what's happening when in the process of pooing or weeing; and that he can give you at least a few minutes warning that he's about to go. Waiting for the right time will almost always make it an easier process. In fact, some parents find that minimal interven-tion is required – some children are happy to take themselves off to the potty when they need to and virtually 'toilet train' themselves.

It's worth noting that boys tend to toilet train later than girls, for reasons that aren't completely clear. And night-time dryness is something that will usually come much later – sometimes not until school age.

Crissy says: Potty training can be a stressful time, but by far the most successful approach is when parents have realistic expectations and tackle the whole business with patience and understanding. Despite what you may have heard, the age at which your child becomes potty trained is no reflection on their future intelligence or ability, and at the end of the day your child will master potty training when he's physiologically, psychologically and emotionally ready and not before. No matter what strategies, tricks or bribery you choose to employ, the biggest single factor in the success or failure of potty training is you, and when potty training really becomes a contentious issue for a child it's often because parents could be handling things a little better. If potty training's turning into a nightmare, with you feeling furious and your little one reduced to tears, just call a halt to the proceedings, give yourself a break for a month or so and then choose a relatively relaxed non-stressful time to try again. Forcing your child to sit on the potty against his will, getting visibly angry or upset or punishing him when he's had an accident can create anxiety around using the potty and in the long run is more likely to cause him to rebel or even to start withholding his bodily waste. This can lead to a vicious circle as it will become painful to go and therefore he'll be even less likely to try.

Some toddlers are quite possessive of their poo and reluctant to see it flushed away, and some are fearful of the flush itself, the splashing sound their wee makes in the potty or the risk they might fall into or off their throne. Take time to listen to your child. Find out how he really feels about using the potty and make sure he understands what is and isn't expected of him. Your child may be frightened of the bathroom itself, so make sure it becomes a welcoming and familiar place. Buy some new bath toys or bubble bath and designate a special towel just for him, pop his teddy or a favourite doll on the loo while he's on the potty, and make sure you stay with him for support and entertainment. He should only be trying for short periods at first so there won't be time to nip off and finish the dishes. Make sure, too, that he's comfy and that the potty is stable. Potty chairs are generally more comfortable and have the added security of handles and a back rest. Kids need to have their feet firmly on the ground in order to control the muscles they need to go and also to feel safe, so if they're on the loo you'll need a foot rest and, if possible, a child seat. Take the pressure off and reward your child with praise for his efforts rather than for his achievements so he knows that in these early days it's more about trying than succeeding.

What the netmums say

It's potty time

Elliot was two years and one month when he started running off while we were playing and popping himself on the potty to poo! I'd introduced him to it when he was about eighteen months, encouraging him to sit on it when I went to the loo, and talking lots about wees and poos. I made sure it was always around, and accessible for him. Six months on he's dry during the day, and dry most nights, too.
Jeni-Ann from Darwen, mum to Elliot, two

I bought a potty at around eighteen months. We had it alongside all his toys, and talked about what we did on the potty. Mummy even gave a rough demonstration! Eventually, at almost three, my son was going to a childminder with a friend who was potty trained, and they took to going to the toilet at the same time. From then on my son took to it immediately and had no accidents, because he was ready to do it. I think if you push a child when they aren't ready, you're likely to hit problems. My advice is to stay relaxed, plan for when you're out and about – and make sure you always know where the nearest toilet is!
Hayley from Staines, mum to Jay, four

My son was happy to sit on the potty in his clothes, but refused to sit down without them. Then when he was two and a half, he saw one of my friend's boys use the toilet, and asked for the potty when we got home. He was potty trained within a week. My daughter understands what the potty is for, but won't sit down long enough to use it. I will be guided by her and wait until she's ready.
Natasha from Plymouth, mum to Kieran, four, and Livvy, two

Damien was just over two when he told me that he wanted to use the big toilet, and didn't want to wear nappies any more. It was out of the blue and I was thirty-five weeks' pregnant, so the timing wasn't great. He knew best though, and within a week he was

accident-free – with only a short regression when his brother came along. We skipped the potty stage and went straight to the toilet, using a 'two-in-one' toilet seat, which has a small seat for children and a normal seat for adults. I didn't see the point in training to use a potty then when he got the hang of that training him to do something else. He was rewarded with one sweet for a wee, and two for a poo. I also gave lots and lots of praise when he got it right and didn't comment when he got it wrong. A year later, he decided that he didn't want to wear nappies to bed any more – again, I thought there was no way he was ready. But yet again, he knew best, and apart from a handful of occasions, he's been dry ever since. Quinn is now starting to show an interest in using the toilet, so fingers crossed it will be as easy second time round.
Yvonne from Ayr, mum to Damien, four, and Quinn, two

My eldest attempted potty training at about eighteen months and was doing very well, but a few months later her little sister was born and she regressed and would no longer use it. I finally succeeded in getting her potty trained, with a lot of hard work, at two years and eight months. Her younger sister was potty trained at twenty-two months, but I think having an older sibling helped.
Alexis from Camberley, mum to Sophie, four, and Chloe, two

Abby was around two years old and was quite easy to toilet train. At first I put her in pull-ups, until I realised they were too much like a nappy and too comfortable. I think she'd still be in them now if I'd left it up to her! At three and a half, although he initially showed signs about a year ago, and would even occasionally use the potty, my son had not really progressed further. I hadn't pushed it because he's had a speech delay and felt he had enough on his plate with speech therapy, so I left him in nappies. However, five months ago he started using the toilet of his own accord and we've not looked back. He wears pants all day, and is mainly accident-free. He's struggled a bit more with using the potty or toilet for a poo, but also did that recently for the first time. Cue lots of partying on our part!
Steph from Stoke-on-Trent, mum to Abby, seven, and Drew, three

My feeling is that a lot of mums try to potty train their kids too early. The child has to be mentally developed enough to understand when they need to go and physically able to hold it in and get to the potty. My son didn't like the potty at all and insisted on using the toilet. I found a toilet-training seat very useful as he felt he was a 'big' boy using it and it was easier for him to then move on to the toilet properly. Also, reward stickers every time he went really gave him the incentive to keep at it.
Sonia from County Tyrone, mum to Kacey, nine, and Caleb, four

When she started showing the usual signs of being ready for toilet training around eighteen months to two years, I bought my daughter what I called a 'posh potty'! But she was not interested at all; she wouldn't even sit on it. I took the potty upstairs in the bathroom and when I gave her a bath I sat her on it as I dried her and then spent a while singing to her in the hope it would help her go. She did manage it twice. I also introduced a reward chart and for every five wees on the potty, she got a treat. The week she was two and a half, I was off work, so I let her roam around for two days with no nappy on and it worked a treat. When we had to go out for the day I was worried it would undo all the hard work but I just took a potty with me, got her to use it every half hour, and she was dry all day. I told her if she could stay in big-girl pants then I would buy her the doll she wanted, which she did get, and named Tinkle!
Tracy from Bromsgrove, mum to Eva, five

I had two different results from the same approach with my two. My daughter was two years and three months, and we focused on it in a half-term week with chocolate buttons and sticker treats every time she used the potty. We started with puddles round the house and a bit of a battle to sit on the potty when needed but a couple of days later, once she realised what the reward system was all about, we had success. Being my first child, I think I was a bit too potty-led and anxious about accidents, and it took a while to get her on the toilet proper. As for my son, I decided to train him at two years five months, before any of the classic signs had appeared, and again during half term. He did it in the week, jelly

babies being his chosen reward. He went dry through the night at the same time and got on to the toilet proper within a month. I know some people swear by being child-led, but I know my kids and if I'd let my son decide when to do it he'd probably still be in nappies now!
Viv from Melksham, mum to Edith, five, and Alban, three

We started potty training when Tyler was twenty-two months. I was naïve to think that he would be fully toilet trained in a few weeks. I used pull-ups, but wish from the very beginning I had been braver and gone straight into pants, as once we left the pull-ups behind it was so much easier. Pooing was more difficult as he did not like 'performing' in front of anyone, opting for a quiet corner on his own. He's now finally toilet trained and this week has also seen him stand up and aim, and most mornings dry.
Christine from Monkton, mum to Tyler, two

I got a couple of potties and toilet seats when Jadon was twenty months old, as I wanted to take a baby-led approach and give him plenty of time to figure things out. For a few months I just talked about the potty, let him sit on it, read a fun book about it, and had lots of nappy-free time at home. I also talked about it whenever I could, at every nappy change and when I went to the toilet. When he had an accident I cleaned up and talked about poo/wee in the potty and toilet, so he watched and listened to what he was supposed to do. I also sang lots of silly songs so he thought the whole thing was a game. At twenty-six months, he managed to stop a wee then sit on the potty and finish. From then on he was very independent and used the potty whenever we were home and I had let him have some nappy-off time. He was so proud of himself! I kept a nappy on when we were really busy or when we were out. He wouldn't tell me when he needed to go or when he had gone so I had to watch him carefully when we were out at playgroups but after a few months he was happy to use the potty or toilet even when out. It took a while for him to tell me he needs to go, rather than me watching the clock and nagging him to try, but he's now dry all day, and very independent. His little brother has been watching all this and started using the potty a few months ago at nineteen months. They're both really motivated by producing something in the potty or toilet so I've never bothered with rewards. I've been positive, though, and always offered loads of praise.

Ingrid from Warwick, mum to Jadon, three, Caleb, twenty-one months, and Bram, four months

50 What's with the tantrums?

It can come as a bit of a shock when your previously placid little one starts throwing tantrums. One minute she's playing happily, the next she's chucked herself on to the floor in a tear-streaked rage – and all without any apparently good reason. Although perplexing and often tough to cope with, this sort of behaviour is completely normal in toddlers. Tantrums are extremely common in the period known as 'the terrible twos' – but don't be surprised if your little one starts stamping her feet well before her second birthday, or keeps them up well beyond her third. Mostly, tantrums are caused by sheer frustration: your toddler has a fast-developing brain and she's starting to know what she wants in life, but she may not have the language or developmental skills she needs to acquire it – or maybe she's simply been told by you that she can't! At this tender age, disappointment is not easily dealt with: and let's face it, you can't really expect a two-year-old to have much in the way of anger management skills. Sometimes, screaming and shouting about it is the only way she can find to communicate her feelings at the time.

Often you can pre-empt a tantrum with a bit of distraction. But sometimes, there's no avoiding it: when she blows, she blows. Then it's usually a question of battening down the hatches, and waiting for the storm to pass.

What the experts say

Crissy says: Toddlers generally tantrum when they feel frustrated or thwarted in some way. They have no concept as yet of delayed gratification – when they want something, they want it NOW! Being of the confirmed opinion that the world does and should revolve around them, they naturally expect to get their own way and so when you give in to their tantrums it's hardly surprising if they adopt throwing a wobbly as their weapon of choice in their ongoing battle for increased independence. At this age, kids are desperate to gain more control over their lives and to begin making decisions for themselves, but as toddlers are hardly renowned for their sound judgement in these matters they are often denied this autonomy by their parents, which they quite understandably find infuriating. Despite its bad press, anger is an entirely natural emotional response and it's far healthier for your child to be able to express her anger openly than bottling it up. The trouble is that toddlers have yet to develop the level of self-control necessary to rid themselves of all that aggressive energy without resorting to tantrums, and so they'll need you to set them a good example.

When dealing with tantrums, not surprisingly prevention is often the best option, so keep your eyes peeled for signs of a storm brewing – if you're able to distract your child or redirect her focus, all well and good. Take note of your child's principle tantrum triggers, and do your best to avoid them, especially when she's tired or hungry. Make sure you have realistic expectations of your child's behaviour and choose your battles wisely rather than picking up on every single thing you feel she's doing wrong. If you notice her becoming upset, encourage her to share how she's feeling and why, but make it clear that although you understand she may be feeling angry, having a tantrum won't change your mind or get her what she wants. If the situation deteriorates towards a tantrum let her know that you won't discuss the matter further until she's calmed down and then if all else fails step back and leave her to it. The whole point of a tantrum is that it needs an audience so even when you're seething inside or cringing with embarrassment you'll need to stay calm on the outside, and do your best to at least pretend you're oblivious to all the fuss. Stand firm, but resist being drawn into a battle of wills and don't yell, hit back or rough handle her. If you do decide to give in for a quiet life remember you may be buying time now, but in the long run you're making a rod for your own back, so make it a rule never to reward a tantrum or resort to bribery.

When a tantrum really gets out of hand and there's a risk of physical harm you will of course need to step in to defuse the situation. Don't tower over her, but take yourself down to her eye level and talk calmly and quietly. Children will often lower their own volume to hear you. Try to make and to sustain eye contact and aim for respectful empathy rather than personal insults and a good telling-off. Toddlers can frighten themselves with the force of their tantrum and so it may help to contain her fury and make her feel more secure if you soothe her by holding her firmly in your arms until she's calmed down.

Some toddlers are left reeling from anxiety or exhaustion following a tantrum but children vary in what they need so be guided by her. Avoid holding a post mortem after the event, which could be shaming for her: instead offer her the reassurance that you still love her and if it seems welcome, an opportunity to make amends.

One of the most comforting ways of looking at toddler tantrums is to remember that it's actually a good thing when children push the boundaries because it shows they have spirit and are developing exactly as they should be. The reason they act up with you is because they are secure in your love and trust that you won't reject them even when they are behaving badly. Try bearing this in mind the next time you find yourself cringing at the judgemental tuts and sighs in the supermarket queue!

What the netmums say

Toddler wobblers

My son started early with the tantrums. He was frustrated that he couldn't communicate what he wanted, and this would often set him off. After a while I learnt that the best response was simply to put him somewhere safe and let him do his thing. When he was

ready, he would come to me for a cuddle. I know it was far more effective and quicker than trying to talk him out of it. He'd only continue to scream and get frustrated at not being understood.
Hayley from Staines, mum to Jay, four

Charlie still has tantrums. They're worse when he's hungry or tired, but usually they have a direct cause, such as being told 'no' when he wants a biscuit. We let him blow, then talk to him and cuddle him and distract him with something else such as a favourite toy. Fortunately, they're usually at home. When Eve was younger, I recall her having them in public and sometimes having to just pick her up and walk out, leaving a trolley of shopping behind if necessary! You just have to remember that you are in control, not them. Not easy, I know.
Julie from Lichfield, mum to Eve, twelve, Charlie, two, and Amy, seven months

Bethany is just learning her boundaries. Occasionally she will have an all-out meltdown, usually because she's trying to work something out and it's not going well. In this case, I just distract her. If she's being naughty because she wanted something she couldn't have, I tell her once she will go in her cot. That normally sorts it, but if she continues, she goes in her cot for a few minutes to cool off. She's soon back to her sunny self.
Ruth from Newton Abbot, mum to Bethany, seventeen months, and Thomas, five months

At fifteen months, my daughter is already throwing tantrums – usually if she is tired but also if I say no to something she wants, or if she is frustrated. I wasn't expecting to get tantrums this early, but I guess every child is different. I try to avoid them by telling her what will be happening next and trying to get her to take part in choices, but sometimes they can't be avoided. During these times, I either ignore her and allow the tantrum to run its course or (if we are in a public place) pick her up and carry on as normal. Generally she's absolutely gorgeous and I guess these tantrums are just her way of telling me what she wants or her frustrations, while she can't express them in another way.
Becks from London, mum to Eloise, fifteen months

Rory started having tantrums at the age of one. Usually they involved him finding something hard and repeatedly hitting his head on it. Obviously I was concerned and asked my health visitor, but having been told 'he will grow out of it', the only thing we can do is look away. He seems to like an audience and stops if he is ignored. We'll do anything to try and prevent a tantrum when one seems to be brewing, from distraction to bribery, as they are pretty scary!

Jenna from Leeds, mum to Paige, three, and Rory, eighteen months

My son is fast perfecting the art of the tantrum already. He started walking at fourteen months, and I think he gets frustrated if he's stopped from going where he wants to go or doing what he wants to do. I find that bribery works if you want them to do something but it won't stop unwanted behaviour. And routine helps: tantrums are less likely if he's been fed, watered, changed, has slept, and had a good run around. I try to be consistent and not to give mixed messages, as I imagine it would be frustrating if something is allowed one day but not the next. And if one's brewing, I offer lots of distraction. When one does erupt (and sometimes there's just no preventing it) I try to be calm, and offer a way out without 'giving in'. Don't make it into a battle, is my advice. If you feel you're becoming wound up, take a few minutes out. When the storm has passed, offer a big cuddle and tell them, 'I love you.'

Lucy from Peterborough, mum to Isaac, sixteen months

My wee guy is pretty good when it comes to tantrums. They're few and far between, but when they do happen, he's always tired. That combined with not getting his own way usually sets him off. If it's not yet bedtime and he wants a feed but I tell him no, because I know if he nurses he'll fall asleep too early, that usually starts a tantrum. Another thing that sets him off is if he wants a bit of something that has dairy in it but he can't have it, because of his allergy. I make sure I have a stock of dairy-free buttons, ready-salted crisps, grapes and strawberries at all times, just in case. As for tiredness before bedtime, distraction normally works a treat.

Marianne from Uddingston, mum to William, twenty-two months

Mine all hit the so-called 'terrible twos' at thirteen months – and my seven-year-old has yet to entirely outgrow them! With Sian I could usually stop a tantrum with food and drink (and actually, even now her strops tend to be blood-sugar-related). Beth is more stubborn and nothing seemed to stop them. Rick had one only recently, in the supermarket. I ended up moving him to a corner and ignoring him, and twenty minutes later he climbed back into the pushchair, of his own accord. But not before I'd been stared at by folks! One old gentleman doing his shopping seemed to sympathise, and stopped to smile.

Geina from Feltham, mum to Sian, seven, Beth, five, and Rick, two

We never got bad tantrums from my son so, boy, did my daughter come as a shock. Beginning not long after her first birthday, she would have the most horrendous tantrums. She would scream and throw herself backwards, bashing her head on whatever was behind her, and when that wasn't effective she would sit cross-legged and deliberately bash her forehead on the floor to get some reaction. We used to mainly ignore it as long as she wasn't in any danger, but it was hard when it was that extreme. Once she did it in the supermarket and I walked away and got a mouthful from some woman who didn't approve! If we were somewhere quiet like a restaurant and she did it, one of us would just pick her up and carry her out. At home, we would take her to her room to calm down where she would kick walls and doors and it would take ages to calm down. Sometimes she'd get so worked up, she would almost make herself sick. But it was pointless trying to cuddle her to calm her down, as that would only make her worse. Now she's three she has a lovely temperament. She still has her moments, but I'm relieved to say we got past that particular stage.

Sarah from Camberley, mum to Judd, eight, and Sian, three

Useful addresses

General advice and support for new mums

Netmums
The UK's largest parenting website, offering advice and support, information, online forums and local meet-up groups throughout the country.
Web: www.netmums.com

National Childbirth Trust (NCT)
Offers support, advice and friendship during pregnancy, childbirth and early parenthood. Valley cushions (inflatable cushions that offer relief when sitting if you are sore after birth) and breast pumps for hire.
Postnatal Line: 0300 330 0773
Web: www.nct.org.uk

Bliss
UK charity offering support and advice for parents of premature babies.
Support helpline: 0500 618 140
Web: www.bliss.org.uk

Home-Start
Nationwide charity that offers practical support and friendship to families in need through a network of parent volunteers.
Information line: 0800 068 6368
Web: www.home-start.org.uk.

Family Lives (formerly Parentline)
Registered charity offering support to anyone parenting a child of any age.

Helpline: 0808 800 2222
Web: www.familylives.org.uk

Healthy Start
Government scheme providing needy families with vouchers for free milk, fruit and veg, formula and vitamin supplements.
Web: www.healthystart.nhs.uk.

NHS Direct
Medical advice from qualified staff available over the telephone. NHS Direct serves England and Wales.
Tel: 0845 4647
Web: www.nhsdirect.nhs.uk

NHS24
Medical advice from qualified staff available over the telephone, serving Scotland.
Tel: 08454 242424
Web: www.nhs24.com

Cry-sis
Support for families with excessively crying, sleepless and demanding babies.
Helpline: 08451 228 669
Web: www.cry-sis.org.uk

Breastfeeding

Breastfeeding NHS
National breastfeeding helpline: 0300 100 0212
Web: www.breastfeeding.nhs.uk

National Childbirth Trust
Breastfeeding Line: 0300 330 0771
Web: www.nct.org.uk

Association of Breastfeeding Mothers
Counselling helpline: 08444 122 949
Web: www.abm.me.uk

Breastfeeding network
Supporter line: 0300 100 0210
Web: www.breastfeedingnetwork.org.uk

La Leche League
Helpline: 0845 120 2918
Web: www.laleche.org.uk

The Baby Cafe
Charitable trust that runs a network of local drop-in centres for breastfeeding mums.
Web: www.thebabycafe.co.uk

Multiple births

Twins and Multiple Births Association (TAMBA)
Freephone 'twinline': 0800 138 0509
Web: www.tamba.org.uk

The Multiple Births Foundation
Tel: 0208 383 3519
Web: www.multiplebirths.org.uk

Twins UK
Organisation offering information and support for families with twins, triplets or more.
Expert advice line: 01670 856996
Web: www.twinsuk.co.uk

Safe sleeping

Foundation for the Study of Infant Deaths (FSID)
Charity working to prevent cot death, offer safe sleep advice and give support to bereaved parents.
Free helpline: 0808 802 6868
Web: www.fsid.org.uk

Safety

Child Accident Prevention Trust (CAPT)
Safety advice and information line: 020 7608 7364
Web: www.capt.org.uk

Royal Society for the Prevention of Accidents (RoSPA)
Web: www.rospa.com

Postnatal depression

Association for Postnatal Illness (APNI)
Telephone helpline and information for sufferers and healthcare professionals as well as a network of volunteer supporters who have themselves experienced postnatal illness.
Helpline: 020 7386 0868
Web: www.apni.org

Perinatal Illness UK
Charity offering support to anyone suffering from emotional or psychological difficulties during pregnancy or after birth.
Web: www.pni-uk.com

Depression Alliance
Works to relieve and prevent depression, providing information and support.
Information pack request line: 0845 123 2320
Web: www.depressionalliance.org

House of Light
Charity providing support, information and advice for women suffering from PND and their families.
Helpline: 0800 043 2031
Web: www.pndsupport.co.uk

Relationships

Relate
Relationship advice and counselling, sex therapy, workshops, mediation, consultations and support offered face to face, by telephone and through the web.
Tel: 0300 100 1234
Web: www.relate.org.uk

The Parent Connection
Website offering relationship advice to parents.
Web: www.theparentconnection.org.uk

Weaning

British Dietetic Association
Professional association for registered dietitians in the UK. Its website is a

useful source of information about weaning and other dietary matters.
Web: www.bda.uk.com

Baby Led Weaning
Information, recipes and forums for parents keen to try weaning the baby-led way.
Web: www.babyledweaning.com

Annabel Karmel
Website of the popular baby and toddler food expert, offering recipe ideas.
Web: www.annabelkarmel.com

Allergy UK
Support and information for people with allergies and intolerances.
Tel (helpline): 01322 619898
Web: www.allergyuk.org

Kids' Allergies
Lots of useful information and advice about children and allergies.
Web: www.kidsallergies.co.uk

Work and childcare

Working Families
Organisation offering advice and information on all aspects of working families' lives, including tax credits, childcare and legal rights.
Parents and carers helpline: 0800 013 0313
Web: www.workingfamilies.org.uk.

Daycare Trust
Charity working to promote and provide information about affordable childcare.
Web: www.daycaretrust.org.uk

Index